MANIFESTO
FOR A
CANCER PATIENT

Copyright © 2017 Colleen Huber, NMD
ISBN: 978-0-692-98347-8

Medical Choice Editions

Preface

To state the obvious, before diagnosis and after remission or cure, "cancer patient" does not apply to the person. A cancer patient may well request that you take away each of those words altogether and permanently, which seems to be a fair request, because life begins for us without either of those words, and continues preferably without either of them, but more importantly, because such a label seems misapplied to a thinking person who is deciding the best course of medical treatment. Before and after a cancer journey, but especially during a person's brief vestment with the words "cancer patient," I hope this book will serve as a useful manifesto and manual.

Many of the people whom I have met during the last eleven years in my naturopathic cancer clinic feared or expected cancer in their own future, perhaps due to family history, and many never expected it at all. But almost everyone seems surprised at the suddenness of the diagnosis, with abrupt change in status, from freely independent thinker, in control of one's destiny, to suddenly cast in scripted institutional theater, cast in an unwanted role, unable to assert choices as before, and having one's preferences challenged by others.

The purpose of this book is to focus attention on the sovereignty of the individual who receives a cancer diagnosis. What is personal sovereignty? The sovereignty of nations is commonly recognized, but what of individuals? Libertarians among others understand well the concept of, and need for, personal liberties, and vote accordingly. 'Don't tread on me' asserts where a larger entity must defer to the self-determination of a smaller entity, or the boundary of where governance ends, and where my self-determination begins. But where is patient advocacy and the libertarian primer for the novice in the oncology clinic?

I pause my diatribe there, because I first owe the reader a reason for entertaining my views through the length of this book on the rights of cancer patients. I am a Naturopathic Medical Doctor, my medical education being from a 4-year naturopathic medical school, Southwest College of Naturopathic Medicine in Tempe, AZ. My license to practice medicine in Arizona is number 06-948, a small number due to the small number of licensed naturopathic physicians in my state when I was first licensed in 2006. Most doctors who treat cancer don't have much to do with alternative medicine. Most alternative doctors don't see a lot of cancer patients. I do both, and my clinic is dedicated to that pursuit full-time over the last eleven years.

The way that I treat cancer patients is within the laws of the US and of Arizona, but very much different from conventional oncology. Our clinic has, I believe, pioneered a multi-faceted cancer-disrupting protocol, because fighting cancer in multiple ways simultaneously is a stronger, more permanent way to defeat cancer than with one or a few medications, as I will argue at length throughout the book. I treat cancer patients with intravenous nutrients, exercise and such. 'And such' includes quite a bit more, varying a lot among individuals. I have had better success than in conventional oncology clinics, and I demonstrate the success that we have had in detail in Chapter 7.

Regarding the reading experience of this book, I must advise the reader that Chapter 7, Defeating cancer requires more than one treatment method, is a long and tedious bore. Chapter 6 and Chapter 8 are fairly dreary also. I wrote those as articles over the last several years, because in my line of work, one must document everything in daily charting of medical notes, both successful and failing results, because of relentless and intense scrutiny. It seems to me that the skeptics whom I encounter are more numerous or at least more boisterous than those who already entrust me to do the best for them and more numerous by far than those who simply approach the topic of natural treatments for cancer with an unbiased, open mind. Chapter 7 began as a reprint and is now an expansion of my article of the same name, first written in 2009 and updated each year since. Those who wish to skim over that chapter will understand the gist of it in the first few pages of Chapter 7. On the other hand, for those who wish to dig deeper in the data, you are welcome to it; all of the information that we had up to 2014 is reported there. Therefore, one may draw conclusions that our clinic has not yet looked for, such as comparing the remission rate of our colorectal cancer patients who had surgery with those who did not, for example, or the remission rate of the pancreatic cancer patients who avoided sweetened foods with those who did not, as another example.

One might wonder why we stopped this detailed compilation of data in 2014. Why not continue? Before 2014, I had met every patient who came to us with a biopsied cancer. Now our clinic is large enough that I have only met about one fourth of the patients who currently come to us. These days our follow-through does not necessarily continue with the same doctor through all of a patient's treatments. I would like to think that the left hand is as in touch with the right hand now as it was in the earlier years of our clinic, but to tell the truth, we have slipped a bit in that regard with our growing size. Diligent, daily chart notes are not adequate to pursue all follow-through, because the patients' stories and reported feelings and observations of vitality and wellbeing do not always begin and end with the same doctor, and are harder to track now because of that.

Therefore, even though it is a little dated, I include Chapter 7 here in the manuscript, with the earlier chapters as prefatory to it, because the data reported in that chapter is the basis for the conclusions in, not only the paper, but further study and reflection at our clinic. That reflection and the lessons learned from our experiences in the clinic has given rise to this book. The Defeating Cancer paper has been published and updated annually since 2009 on our website NatureWorksBest.com, although it was also presented as the keynote speech at the Euro Cancer Summit in 2015,[1] and in the Journal of Cancer Science and Therapy.[2]

Let the reader be forewarned: the reason that Chapter 7 is *very* tedious is that it reports, anonymously, all the studied results of all cancer patients – the successful as well as not so successful, without excluding even one patient who spent at least two weeks in our care – from the beginning of our clinic through 2014 for the main data table. Then yearly updates of parts of that information, rather than the whole, were more feasible to gather and study. Therefore, there is an enormous amount of data. The casual reader may want to skim the tables in that chapter to get the gist. The more diligent reader, however, can take that data to draw conclusions of their own, which we have never analyzed: For example, how much more successful have we been with say breast cancer than each of the other cancers? How many times per week must one exercise to have at least an 80% chance of going into remission? A diligent reader has all the tools in Chapters 6, 7 and 8 to be able to calculate answers to such questions and unimaginably many more questions. We invite the dissection and analysis, as it will help to enrich general knowledge of how humans, now and in the future, best defeat cancer.

As Keynote Speaker, I presented that paper to the Euro Cancer Summit in Valencia, Spain, November, 2015. One can search that event online for the abstract. It can also be found here:

http://cancer.global-summit.com/europe/abstract/2015/defeating-cancer-requires-more-than-one-treatment-method-an-8-year-retrospective-case-series-using-multiple-nutritional-and-herbal-agents-2014-update

Chapter 8 is another difficult chapter in that it is reprinted from a medical journal, and therefore has more scientific jargon than the casual reader may wish to bother reading. That chapter, Glycemic restriction in cancer patients, was first published in Cancer Strategies Journal, Spring 2014, Volume 11, Issue 2. That journal is no longer in publication.

For both Chapters 7 and 8, the conclusion at the end is: an extraordinarily high success rate against cancers in humans was achieved with natural treatments, primarily intravenous nutrients and a dietary intervention. These results have surpassed those of chemotherapy clinics to the best of our knowledge. In fact, we have not seen any better results from any cancer clinic anywhere in the world that publishes its results with all patients, as we do. Nor has any of our patients alerted us to the presence of a more successful clinic. Most of our patients are diligent individuals who study all they can about their particular cancers and the treatments available for them. We are grateful for the opportunity we have to help advance the knowledge of cancer and how to defeat its presence and progress through the body. We are appreciative of our role in safe and effective cancer treatment, and we present the data in Chapters 7 and 8, not only to show what we have already examined, but so that the reader may also take any part of that raw data and determine what further lessons lie within it, so that we may all move forward more productively in the best possible direction.

Acknowledgements

Naturopathic physicians have twice as many classroom hours and twice as many courses in medical school as MDs and DOs. (See endnote 10). None of our reported data would be possible, and none of the formidable results obtained at the clinic, if it weren't for the outstanding physicians and staff with whom I am privileged to work:

Dr. Kenneth Lashutka, who has been a bulwark of common sense and excellent medical judgment, in the face of all kinds of patient circumstances and the largest variety of different kinds of cancer that I imagine a doctor could possibly face.

Dr. Debbie Rogalla, who is the most thoroughly educated physician of any kind I have ever met. Over the past decade, Dr. Rogalla has traveled extensively to learn from many of the top minds in medicine. Her vast knowledge is a great treasure that we are privileged and honored to welcome at our clinic.

Dr. Nick Johnson, who brings his knowledge and experience in nuclear medicine as well as a naturopathic physician to our fortunate clinic. Dr. Johnson manages to balance his considerable knowledge with deep compassion, endearing him to patients as well as to the staff.

Our wonderful nursing staff and medical assistants, who are truly fabulous in their jobs, in their compassion and caring for the patients, as well as their expertise in their field.

Our incredible Office Manager, Lori, whom I have learned to appreciate as the voice and face of the clinic, often the first voice of warmth, good sense and compassion from the medical field to patients newly diagnosed with cancer.

Thank you also to my husband and to my child, who are very patient and supportive of my work.

Thank you to our incredible website staff, Nick, Chris and Alexa.

Thanks also to María, Steve and Mary, and a very humble and sincere thank you to the patients whom it has been our privilege and honor to serve.

Deepest gratitude of all goes to our favorite mentor physician, Dr. Kenneth Proefrock, who has taken the standard of a brilliant medical mind up to a level that is world-class, inspiring and supersedes known precedent among the living, to the best of my knowledge.

MANIFESTO

FOR A
CANCER PATIENT

Colleen Huber, NMD

Medical Choice Editions

Table of Contents

13

Part 1
Manifesto for a Cancer Patient

Introduction

What choices do cancer patients have?

I have an eleven-year old naturopathic cancer clinic in Tempe, Arizona. To even say that a decade ago invited disdain from all sides, except from patients and their family and friends who happened to be glad for our existence, as a lone outpost of alternative medicine in an otherwise bleak landscape inhabited by cancer patients in our time, a landscape where even those clinics that so persistently advertise their "natural treatments for cancer" soon reveal their fine print to newcomers: There is a catch to the natural treatments. You see, you get the natural treatments, only if you also agree to chemotherapy. I'll discuss this particular trap more later.

In contrast, at our clinic we never once insisted on chemotherapy or radiation to any cancer patients. It has always been our policy to pledge, and to do our best to deliver, our best efforts, regardless of the other choices our patients made in their treatment. In fact, I tell new patients, "I owe you my best efforts, whether you choose to also have chemotherapy, or you choose

15

not to have it." It is not my place to make such a life-altering decision for the patient. Regardless of which course or combination of treatments the patient chooses, I want the best outcome, and I'll do my best to help eliminate that person's cancer.

So when new patients found in our clinic that what you see is what you get, and no you do not have to have chemotherapy, they and their empathetic family members tended to feel relieved to say the least. This does not include all family and friends of patients, because almost every patient came in with a story of one or more hypervigilant and dogmatic family members who would insist that the patient follow every dictate of the chemotherapy oncologist, or who would insist that the patient either shun or embrace natural treatments for cancer. So often the patient, already weakened and stressed to the breaking point by their disease, would be further shoved and yanked as a rope in a tug of war between warring sides of their family. Patients complained to me that although it was certainly possible to ruin an otherwise peaceful Thanksgiving dinner by discussing politics, likewise such an occasion can be ruined by a debate between pharmaceutical advocates and pharmaceutical skeptics. Or if you prefer, the drug nuts versus the health nuts. Enough rancor to make anyone of us nuts, particularly someone whose health is already frail. Later I'll also discuss why cancer patients are not likely to fight the most belligerently of all family members, even back in better days when they were feeling well.

But first, I should let you know what it was like to practice naturopathic medicine with cancer patients in the bad old days. Back in 2006 when I started my

16

clinic, it was commonly thought that chemotherapy was a necessary and helpful treatment, the main treatment even, for almost all cancers, unthinkable to simply decide not to have it.   Not an option.   Oncologists were known to tell patients: "You're sick anyway, so why should you care about some side effects from chemo? Besides, hair grows back." (That is, for the lucky minority who survived their full prescribed course of chemotherapy treatments.)

Immunotherapy had not yet gained much traction, and even though cancer care was going in much more interesting directions in Europe and in Asia at that time, the US media never discussed such phenomena except in a few dismissive sentences. US universities and other US research institutes generally look disdainfully at research coming from abroad, even though there is more evidence of Pharma corruption of US medical research than of research originating elsewhere in the world.[3]   Even in cancers where chemotherapy had already been proven ineffective, it was "standard of care."

In such an environment, nearly every naturopathic physician who had anything to do with cancer acted as adjunct therapists to chemo oncologists. And even when they knew better, many of these naturopathic physicians insisted on their patients' having chemotherapy and radiation as a prerequisite to natural treatments, which very unfortunately forced patients to undergo toxic and often fatal conventional treatments against their will. A number of these naturopathic physicians alleged (falsely) to naturopathic medical students that to do otherwise was illegal, while newer voices in the naturopathic community began to protest the chemo cartel and its corrupting influence in our naturopathic medical profession. That cartel argued to state and national professional associations and regulatory authorities that they should be the only naturopathic physicians permitted to work with cancer patients. Due to top-down hierarchical structure and a clubby, cartel-like culture, those physicians had all taken an exam that they wrote. They argued not only that they should be the only naturopathic physicians allowed to treat cancer patients, but that their dogmatic views on how to treat cancer patients should be the only ones allowed to prevail.

Fortunately, as it turned out, they did not prevail, and other naturopathic physicians may still treat cancer patients, and likely will continue to be able to do so, and more importantly, cancer patients are no longer universally forced to endure chemotherapy - all due to a couple of timely, and very obscure, moves on the political chessboard, which I will discuss later.

In the late aughts, there were generally only two options available to cancer patients in the United States:

1. (For the vast majority): Follow precisely the instructions of the chemotherapy oncologist (or medical oncologist, as they like to call themselves). You only get this treatment for your cancer: chemotherapy (almost always), radiation treatment (frequently offered) and surgery (IF your tumor burden is operable, and very often only as a bribe after you've been forced to begin chemotherapy.) That's it. No other options. Step onto the conveyor belt, and

slide into the maws of the cancer machine. We are about to get started with you.

OR

2. (For the more fortunate few): Do all of the above without protest, you may try some dietary and supplement recommendations to help you tolerate your chemotherapy better. Terms such as "naturopathic oncologist" have been confusing for the public. Because some of these physicians simply offered natural treatments only for the purpose of palliating symptoms of cancer, and signs and symptoms of chemotherapy toxicity, such naturopathic physicians served only as assistants to medical oncologists, trying to mop up the disastrous health conditions caused by the latter's very toxic treatments. Very unfortunately, such physicians could have chosen to use therapies that were themselves adequate to eliminate cancer, but far too many of them chose not to, or perhaps they chose not to publicize that that was what they were doing. This made the cancer patient doubly unfortunate, already weakened by a life-threatening disease, then further having to sort through the confusing role of the health care practitioners who helped to palliate cancer symptoms and chemotherapy side effects, versus those of us naturopathic physicians who focused our practice on cancer-disrupting, cancer-destroying, cancer-inactivating nutrients and herbs. It is possible, and evident from public statements at naturopathic medical conferences at the time, that alliances with conventional oncology were

due to a desire to be accepted in that realm, and perhaps to taste some of the tremendous flow of money through that industry. A desire not to rock the boat with the chemotherapy oncologists kept such doctors submissive to the demands of the much stronger and larger chemotherapy industry, even to the point of placing those interests above those of cancer patients.

One such intrigue involved an especially notorious transaction, behind closed doors to negotiate with power brokers to remove some of the most effective anti-cancer nutrients out of the scope of naturopathic medical practice, in one of the states where naturopathic medicine is licensed. While the worst of the perpetrators no longer have political power at this time, none were prosecuted. A complaint was made to that state's naturopathic medical board about the loss of these nutrients, and the need to have those substances restored to the naturopathic scope of practice. Fortunately, the substances in question were restored to the scope of practice, and they are again available to cancer patients. I will discuss this event and those substances more at length in the future, but am currently being pressured not to say too much. However, now many other witnesses are as familiar as I am with the events that transpired, and it is only a matter of time before one of them reveals to the public the details of that disgraceful transaction.

Not surprisingly, the general public found the above two choices in cancer treatment to be appallingly inadequate, unsatisfactory and unworthy of the 21st century in the developed world. As Kenneth Proefrock, NMD says, In the US, a country that boasts of its liberties and many choices of lifestyle and destiny for its lucky citizens, you basically have two choices: mashed potatoes or mashed potatoes. However, he points out, those with a long memory can remember other choices that have been available to Americans over time, but that have been taken away, and that "the most subversive thing in America is a long memory." But what is the purpose of a long memory other than to guide our understanding of the times that we now live in? Winston Churchill may have given the best explanation of why a long memory is such a powerful tool: "The farther back you can look, the farther forward you are likely to see." Naturopathic physicians value medicine from all over the world and throughout all history. 5,000 year old traditional Chinese medicine, for example, is not simply quaint folklore, but rather an enduring medicine of universal applicability and value.

Is it hard to believe that medicinal substances have been taken away from the American people and our physicians? At one time, before the 1970s, Americans had access to extract of apricot seeds, commonly called laetrile or vitamin B17 or amygdalin. However, when it was found in the 1970s, by Drs. Moss and Sugiura at Sloan Kettering Institute in New York, to reduce or eliminate tumors in lab mice, it was then outlawed by the FDA, restored in a US District Court, appealed, overturned, and repeatedly batted around judicially with reversals so dizzying that it rivals the twisted, zigzagging legal path in our time of medical marijuana.

Thus, naturopathic physicians have a responsibility to our patients to have a very long memory. Many of the most effective medications in history are from the plant world, with which our ancestors were far better acquainted than are contemporary Americans. Those helpful plant medicines enabled each and every generation of our ancestors to live through their reproductive years and to raise their children, without which success – in every single previous generation without exception - we would not be here. Epigenetic changes in the human species at various places and times, have further co-evolved us with the plant kingdom, so that plant molecules have the most effective key-in-lock effect in our metabolism.

On the other hand, the contemporary alternative offered at nearly every street corner, every television and magazine, are the petrochemical nostrums, aka pharmaceuticals, which have much less use and function in the human body due to their dissimilar nature to the molecules in our own body, much less molecular similarity with us to be able to do a proper job of healing. However, by sheer toxic assault on the body, they can certainly knock out a symptom now and then, even if only replacing the awareness of it with an even more dire symptom, known as a side effect.

The public has always realized this to one extent or another. MD worship is finally starting to wane in the US with the ongoing decline and demise of the WW2 generation and some of the boomers. Health food stores that once were small boutiques with a small but loyal clientele, are now popping up with large parking lots to accommodate an ever growing and more appreciative consumer base. Gyms have been increasing in number and membership.[4] As the casual observer can appreciate the quality of movement and fitness of that consumer base, the appeal of the pharmacies and their products begin to wane. Common-sense values of quality food and exercise over pharmaceutical remedies may account for much of this demographic shift. At this writing, Amazon, the 4th largest corporation on the planet by market capitalization,[5] has just purchased Whole Foods, the largest natural health corporation, and we will see where that takes this particular market trend. So as the previous generations' peculiar deification of the medical doctor comes to be seen for the dead-end cult that it is, the public opens its attention to alternatives for their own health and that of their families.

Although the alternatives to conventional medicine are not formally offered to Americans – What do you MEAN you would rather not have this vaccine? You're getting it now. Roll up your sleeve! – we as a people have the faintest thread of a memory of a time when we actually asserted our rights and declared our sovereignty over our own individual destiny. – No. Actually, I'm NOT going to roll up my sleeve until you show me the package insert for that vaccine with all of the side effects in ALL of the fine print! - And many of us can remember at least one ancestor, and maybe even a parent or a sibling who actually stood up to authority and said "No." No, I will make my own healthcare choices, and if you as a doctor cannot respect that, then I will find another doctor. Or maybe I will go to a naturopath or a chiropractor or an herbalist, but I will not let you force healthcare decisions on me.

Due to demand then, among naturopathic physicians treating cancer patients, and our professional calling to do the absolute best for our patients that we are capable of doing, as if the patients were our own close family members, a number of us law-abiding but less obedient naturopathic physicians, as well as some very courageous and principled medical doctors dating back earlier, felt compelled to rebel against the dictates of the chemotherapy industry. Clearly, in our every interaction with patients and all other parties, we were required at all times to stay within the confines of state and federal law regarding medical practice. Yet we have been even more strongly compelled by the higher authority of our Hippocratic Oath to First Do No Harm. This is an oath that new doctors from both conventional medical schools as well as from naturopathic medical schools must swear to at our graduation from medical school.

The public in general, and cancer patients in particular, have a right to receive the least toxic, least harmful treatments that will work to overcome their condition. There are naturopathic physicians, and I am honored to be among them, who pledge allegiance above all to the best interests of our patients, and as long as we stay within the confines of the law, we will place those primary interests of our patients at all times above the interests of any industry or any old fossils club. We have to make that choice every single day on the job. And we will confidently and steadfastly defend this stance in any court of law any time if challenged on it. In fact, there is one motto that has enabled the continued existence of my clinic over the objections of the Fossils Club, and I apologize in advance to those with delicate sensibilities: You want me to cease to exist? You and what army?

There is a way of asking that question, using a variety of vulgarities popular in US cities, or likely many cities worldwide, such as where I grew up. You and what army? was asked in such assorted colorful ways with off-color words as to establish rights, territory, autonomy. As a public school child, one develops a certain resilience. This resilience is something that I had always taken for granted and thought nothing of at all, until I found myself in more homogenous circles and environments, and there it was strangely lacking. There, in homogenous environments, I did not see so much confidence and bravado as I grew up with, but rather fear and prejudice against outsiders permeating isolated and homogeneous cultural subgroups. These fears seemed to me unfounded.

If such a discussion begins to sound like a digression into sociology, then I'll explain the relevance. Not every personality type would have been comfortable pursuing the kind of work that I do. There are many, probably a majority, who would perceive unacceptable risk in the unthinkable act of 'rocking the boat.' In other words, in order to break outside of a very rigid envelope, to stretch a popular expression, it takes someone who is willing to undergo some personal risk. Yet the risk is more apparent than real, and my clinic was very likely to succeed in our goal of doing right by cancer patients, as long as we practiced within the confines of the law and placed the patients' best interests as primary. Cancer patients, with their very survival at imminent risk, now have no need for the fussy pretensions and business as usual practices and dogma of inadequate cancer treatments such as chemotherapy.   They need something to work correctly for them, the best possible cancer treatments available on the planet, and they need it now, and no thank you, they do not need to wait years for a clinical trial to get underway. If they place their trust in me to save them from death, the very least I can do for them is to match that trust with my courage to give them my best efforts without waiting for approval from old school dogmatists.

Even in 2015 to 2016, when a number of alternative cancer doctors suddenly met with mysterious deaths,[6] it was as if the hydra grew ten more heads, and we did not even consider stopping our work. The result of that particular carnage was that it made the public more aware of natural treatments for cancer, and it strengthened the defenses, surveillance, networks and legal studies of alternative health care practitioners. When cancer patients become aware of better treatment than World War I and II chemical warfare, aka chemotherapy, and when they and their families demand it, rest assured that alternative or naturopathic cancer doctors will be available to meet this need throughout the world. And we are stronger than we ever were, and more numerous.

This is not simply a demand and supply relationship, although labor and business economics dictate that when a job needs to be filled, applicants will arrive. But even more strongly, when lives are at stake, innocent lives of cancer patients, and the potential devastating grief of their dear loved ones are before us, the doctor - who was conscious and inspired by his or her oath at medical school graduation – where we all pledged this - to First Do No Harm and to do best by the patient – that doctor then feels *compelled* and feels *driven* to do everything in human ability to get that patient well, within the confines of the law.

So much has changed over the past decade. A past US president has managed and overcome his cancer through newly developed immunotherapy rather than chemotherapy. There are oncologists who have admitted publicly that it is just a matter of time before chemotherapy will be eventually discarded as safer and more effective treatments for cancer are developed and put into use. Naturopathic physicians are more and more willing to rely on their education and training and best interests of their patients in determining treatment protocols, and no longer so vulnerable as before to pressures from mainstream oncology or other critics. And finally, "naturopathic oncologist" no longer means simply an assistant to a chemotherapy oncologist, but at least, for an increasing number of physicians, is true to the name: One who uses the most effective natural treatments with cancer patients in their fight against cancer, in accordance with naturopathic principles, considering the whole person, the cause of their disease, and teaching how to live in a healthier way, that is a way that is functionally efficient and compatible with vitality and longevity.

But best yet, by far the best, patients themselves are becoming better informed, and more assertive, more willing to defend their right to seek the best treatments available, and have more and far better options in cancer treatment than at any time in history.

Chapter 1

What happens when a person is diagnosed with cancer?

"The Constitution of this Republic should make special provision for medical freedom... Unless we put medical freedom into the Constitution the time will come when medicine will organize into an undercover dictatorship and force people who want doctors and treatment of their own choice to submit to only what the dictating outfit offers."

Benjamin Rush, MD, 1745 – 1813 Colonial Physician and Signer of the United States Declaration of Independence

Chemotherapy oncologists tell a new patient: "Chemotherapy and radiation are the only options available to you. Nothing else will work against your cancer." And then they often say, "Your particular cancer is especially sensitive to chemotherapy. In the kind of cancer that you have, natural treatments do not work."

How do I, a naturopathic oncologist, know that cancer patients routinely hear the above lines? Because regardless of type or stage of cancer, most cancer patients who come to see me tell me that this is what the oncologist told them. I find it strange, and it feeds my cynicism, that most patients have been told that they have the particular type of cancer that chemo would be great for and natural treatments would be bad for.

Then the patient is scheduled to begin chemotherapy treatments promptly. The patient is not offered any of the following:

- The opportunity to take time to look into alternative treatments for cancer,
- The opportunity to get a second opinion from a different doctor,
- The opportunity to simply take time off and think about how to proceed.

The rush job of hurrying as many possible customers into the intake chutes of the cancer machine, the chemotherapy industry, which is a $100 billion dollar industry in the US[7], with an advertising budget in the 100s of millions[8] deprives patients of the opportunity to step back and to assess their options.

In fact, the diagnosis and treatment of cancer are so rushed, that these often happen on consecutive days. The patient is told: "You will begin chemotherapy tomorrow." And, "No you can't postpone chemo, because your insurance is already being billed for it."

Said the spider to the fly.

Naturopathic physicians on the other hand observe a higher standard of medicine than this kind of coercion. Because licensed naturopathic physicians were trained, examined and licensed in both natural and conventional medicine, it is our practice to tell people about BOTH their conventional medicine options AND their natural medicine options. Naturopathic physicians have approximately twice as many classroom hours and twice as many courses in medical schools as medical doctors.[9] This is because we are required to rise to the standards of, and are licensed for, practicing both conventional medicine and natural medicine. This is a much better basis from which to help the patient choose appropriate treatment than someone who was schooled in only one type of medicine.

It is also very important to naturopathic physicians to honor patients' treatment choices. There are naturopathic physicians who look to the American Association of Physicians and Surgeons for their honoring of patient rights[10] and these have been incorporated into some naturopathic physicians' Informed Consent forms, in order to re-affirm patient rights.[11]

- To seek consultation with the physician(s) of their choice;

30

- To contract with their physician(s) on mutually agreeable terms;
- To be treated confidentially, with access to their records limited to those involved in their care or designated by the patient;
- To use their own resources to purchase the care of their choice;
- To refuse medical treatment even if it is recommended by their physician(s);
- To be informed about their medical condition, the risks and benefits of treatment and appropriate alternatives;
- To refuse third-party interference in their medical care

I would therefore like to articulate a naturopathic standard of care for cancer patients, and I would like all cancer patients to be able to assert the following principles with all of their health care providers.

First, it must be recognized that the individual with a new cancer diagnosis faces some of the most difficult decisions of their lives. Cancer patients find themselves immediately surrounded by highly opinionated medical personnel and family members. Why do such treatment decisions belong to the patient instead of to the family or the doctor? I will eagerly answer that question.

Because if we learned anything from World War II, and the subsequent Nuremberg Trials, it is this: That human beings are of free will and sovereignty regarding their own health and decisions pertaining to it. This principle is as self-evident as concepts of equality enshrined in the US Constitution, and in the wisdom of Dr. Rush, the intellectual forebear of conscientious physicians, quoted at the beginning of this chapter, and more specifically regarding individual sovereignty in the Universal Declaration of Human Rights.[12]

This sovereignty of the individual over his or her own health is crystallized in this:

Medical procedures must NOT be forced on people.

It is the right and the responsibility of all physicians to discuss various alternatives for appropriate treatments with their patients, from both conventional and natural medicine as applicable, and to honor patient choices in their health care, with respect shown through word, deed and behavior, and to present treatment choices without coercion or threats or misinformation. Regarding all of those treatment choices, it is incumbent upon others, family and loved ones, to honor patient choices in treatment and in treating physicians.

Only at this juncture, with a fair and respectful physician and home environment, can a cancer patient find the serenity necessary to assess their condition, their prognosis and their options, and to procure the information they need, and to take the time to read the growing amount of material regarding their condition. Only then is the cancer patient able to become best informed and to make the wisest decisions regarding how to proceed, or at least how to begin treatment.

Anybody who stands in the way of those decisions will have a lot to regret, in fact a lifetime of regret, if they carry on their conscience that they bullied or coerced a cancer patient into a possibly fatal course of action.

Let's honor the patient as the wise individual that he or she is, and let's also honor that person's treatment choices. We all owe the cancer patient nothing less than that.

Chapter 2

What do you have a right to expect from a naturopathic oncologist?

The first thing to expect from a naturopathic oncologist is that he or she will listen to you.

Cancer does not arise overnight, and often there is a history of exposure to toxins, radiation or other past assault. Many times even the patient does not know or is not sure what event in their past was most causative of cancer. An initial consult of an hour or more is necessary to try to identify such events, in order to make a plan to reverse damage to the greatest extent possible.

The initial assault leading to cancer varies widely from person to person. However, it is really necessary to try to dig through past history to see if that can be found. Sometimes we meet with auto workers who handled brake pads with asbestos, or people who lived or worked near crop dusters, or under an industrial smokestack. In other cases, there may be extraordinarily high levels of estrogen, or perhaps there were solvents that a person was exposed to. To the extent that these exposures can be reversed, we can get to work on that.

We also do a physical exam, to assess the extent of cancer in the body. We also look at imaging, examining together the CDs or films that patients bring in of their CTs, PET/CTs, MRIs, ultrasounds and x-rays. We piece together a picture of the current tumor burden in the body.

Finally, we talk about treatments. Conventional treatments for cancer are discussed with respect to the individual and his or her tumor burden. There are very different considerations for different parts of the body.

Natural treatments are discussed with the same considerations. Where is the cancer? We fight cancer differently in the lungs than in the prostate, for example. How aggressive is the cancer? Where in the body did it begin? How widespread is it? What is the most precarious or difficult or threatening metastasis? For example, is it wrapped around the aorta? Is it pressing on an eye or ear? Is it pressing against the central bile duct or a ureter? So various suggestions for treatments are given, very often including recommendations for surgery, with all of these considerations. Some patients also consider radiation treatment for an especially precarious tumor burden.

In any case, naturopathic physicians are trained, examined and licensed to practice both conventional and natural medicine. Therefore, naturopathic physicians are uniquely qualified to discuss both your conventional options and your naturopathic options with you. We honor the Patient Bill of Rights, as shown in the Informed Consent on www.NatOnco.org.

Naturopathic oncologists may be found at the following sites:

https://NatOnco.org

https://naturopathicstandards.org/

https://natureworksbest.com/

Chapter 3

Why I became a naturopathic physician

I was raised in a family interested in natural ways of living, choosing whole, natural food over junk food, and looking to nature for medicine when it was needed. All of this seemed to me like a fine way to live, and never seemed to be lacking. We kids grew up strong, healthy with brief bouts of measles, mumps and chicken pox when they each made the rounds of our schools, all very benign and short-term illnesses to healthy kids. Like having a cold, no worse, and you stay home from school a few days, with the added benefit of having a stronger immune system.[13] As we all know, these now rare illnesses have been redrawn and repackaged as the widely-feared bogeymen that effectively hard-sell vaccines. Selling by way of fear works, I suppose, if you can't sell by any more reasonable means. Generally, we played outdoors and indoors for long hours and grew an organic garden long before most people had heard of such a thing, and had really active days outside of school hours.

Against that idyllic and healthy background, Americans had gradually become aware of cancer becoming a relentless and seemingly incurable disease, taking more lives all the time. It seemed to hit as randomly as lightning, with no apparent cause. So my family was horrified to learn in the 1970's that political games in the FDA with backlash in the court system stopped the work of researchers at New York's Sloan Kettering, when they announced a substance, laetrile or vitamin B-17, which could shrink or destroy tumors in mice. As soon as a natural substance was discovered to be effective against cancer, it was made illegal. And that's when the blinders came off. I was now much more interested in natural medicine, and for the first time deeply suspicious of corruption in the institutions most desperately seeking our trust.

America's medical system – no, it goes further - America's lifestyle and culture have been hijacked by an industry that tells you that a doctor is the ultimate arbiter and decision-maker of the health of your whole family. As a result, you no longer feel, or feel confident of, your own autonomy over your own bodies and your own diet and your own decisions. How did our very selves get so thoroughly stolen from our own control?

An article by Mark Hyman, MD, explains better than any other I've seen on the topic of an abysmal problem in the health and lives of Americans: That is, Pharma / government collusion has left the US with the least effective and most dangerous drugs promoted as if they were the only solutions to the health problems of most Americans.[14]

128,000 deaths per year in the US are from "properly" prescribed pharmaceuticals.[15] That's the number reported by doctors and hospitals to the FDA. That's more Americans than died in all of World War I

(116,516) or all of the Vietnam War (90,220).[16]   And that 128,000 is killed each year.   Also, that number does not include deaths from chemotherapy, which are incorrectly called deaths due to cancer.

There are 2.7 million serious, disabling or fatal injuries due to pharmaceuticals each year. And the number of serious adverse events increases over time.[17]

In many cases, such as with "high cholesterol," a problem was alleged, in order to sell a completely unnecessary and very harmful class of drugs as the solution to the non-existent problem. Not surprisingly, that drug class, statins, is the best-selling class of drugs of all time, with the highest revenues. Higher cholesterol is actually correlated with better results against cancer, as Robert Waters, PhD and I showed in 2015.[18]

Why do you never hear about this in the media? Fox's Roger Ailes once told Robert F. Kennedy, Jr. that the major media "gets up to 70% of advertising revenues during non-election years from Pharma."[19] And that is exactly why you will never hear a whisper of a challenge to the tyrannical pharmaceutical industry from anyone but those of us who have a moral obligation to expose such corruption. Fortunately, there are more of us all the time who are speaking out. And more Americans than ever before are looking at the dismal options offered by the conventional medical system and are asking, "Aren't there any better alternatives than this?"

Despite relentless advertising by Pharma, Americans increasingly choose natural medicine and natural lifestyles.[20] 38% of American adults have used some complementary or alternative medicine, although only 43% of those mentioned this to a medical doctor.[21] I look forward to a time when we feel free to choose the health care and lifestyle that we want, without coercion, without artificially induced-fear, and please, for heaven's sake, without endless Pharma commercials such as "Ask your doctor if Quack-o-pill is right for you. Side effects may include brain fog, brainwashing, coma, excessive obedience, and death."

Basically, I became a naturopathic physician, so that people who wanted an alternative to all the damage and carnage above could have a safe sanctuary for their kids and themselves. So that they could have a doctor who would meet their health needs without trying to bully them into unwanted shots and drugs. I wanted, in other words, to be the kind of doctor that my own family and I needed for the rest of our lives.

Chapter 4

Cancer Politics: The Cynical View

I used to wonder if cancer could possibly prey on the most soft-spoken individuals, because of the preponderance of such personality types among the cancer patients at our clinic. When the doctors at my clinic met on initial consult a couple who demonstrated obviously unequal power, with one dictating what will happen, and the other quietly taking orders, it was almost certainly the case that it would be the passive, submissive one that came in with the cancer, rather than the domineering spouse or family member. It was almost as if the disease itself had chosen which type of person to afflict. We saw this again and again. Our doctors and nurses observed this so often and found the pattern so predictable that when a new couple came in, and one was barking at the other, we'd whisper to each other, let me guess which one of those two has the cancer. It was almost as if either a domineering spouse was a resident carcinogen, or a submissive personality pre-disposed the person to cancer, a more predictable and frequently observed risk factor to our observation than even smoking.

However, I no longer think that. Enough strange things have happened to the submissive cancer patients, that I have a more cynical point of view now. I will illustrate with an unfortunate series of events that transpired in the spring of 2016.

A colon cancer patient, whom I'll call Sarah, had achieved remission with our treatments in 2014, without history of chemotherapy or radiation, had an active lifestyle following her bout with cancer, including among many other things, bicycling and some snow shoveling at her home in the mountains. Then she came back in to see me in March 2016. She had sudden onset of lower abdominal pain. On physical exam, I palpated a taut lower abdomen without defined masses. There was tenderness generally through the left and right lower quadrants, as well as more acutely at the site of an abdominal wall hernia that had occurred with her colon resection surgery. Inguinal lymph was not noteworthy. There had been a history of constipation in this patient, but stools had been normal recently. Sarah was pre-menopausal, and this pain was unlike any menstrual cramps she had previously. Specific exams for appendicitis, McBurney's and Rovsing's points were negative, as well as Murphy's point, which tests for appendicitis and gallbladder inflammation, or cholecystitis, respectively, all of those being less likely problems.

There was a possibility of recurrence of colon cancer as the cause of Sarah's pain, but cancer pain is unlikely to have such sudden onset or to worsen so quickly.

An ultrasound may have been adequate to show the cause of the pain, but I knew I could get a lot more information from a MRI. However, health insurance is not so fond of MRIs, and the insurance company dithered, and unfortunately the weekend began without the MRI. On Sunday morning the pain worsened again, and the worried patient and family went to the ER of a large local Phoenix area hospital.

Then, while in her Emergency Room cubicle, no fewer than five doctors walked in and announced to Sarah that her cancer was back, and that she would have to begin chemotherapy and radiation. They had not yet done any imaging or biopsy, yet they announced this diagnosis to the patient. Sarah replied that she wanted to talk to me first, and that she would think about it.

When Sarah called me on Monday morning to tell me what had happened, I said that nothing of that sounded right. By that time, a CT scan had been done in the hospital. Sarah had asked for the disk to look at on her laptop, but was not able to open it. So I hurry over to the hospital with my laptop, as soon as my patient appointments for the day were finished. We open up the CT on my laptop, and all look at it together. What do you know? No cancer visible anywhere! All we saw were two huge fluid-filled ovarian cysts, obliterating each ovary. No wonder the pain was so intense and was worsening so quickly. No wonder no solid mass was apparent to palpation on my physical exam. Ovarian cysts can grow large in a short span of time, quite a bit faster than cancer, and this is likely what happened, since abdominal imaging of several months earlier did not show them at all.

Well, what do you know? Ovarian cysts rather than tumors. Suddenly the doctors who so urgently had to begin chemotherapy and radiation treatments on

Sarah were nowhere to be found. Now the hospital admitted that there was no visible cancer, and oophorectomy (surgery to remove ovaries) was now available. And there was no further mention of chemotherapy.

So Sarah then had the surgery to remove the cysts, as well as the ovaries that were completely blown out by the cysts. Follow-up imaging through early 2017 again confirmed no visible tumor burden.

However, the hospital's mischief was not finished: After the surgery, the hospital pathologist alleged that there were cancer cells in the tissue that was removed from Sarah. So Sarah, now starting to become as cynical as I already am, requests the slides from pathology, so that she and I can study them together.

Once I have the slides in the office, Sarah and I look at a few of them, taking turns examining each field of view at the microscope, but it is very time-consuming to study all fields of some two dozen slides. So after Sarah left, I looked at the rest of them alone. I did not find any cells appearing to be cancer cells on any part of any of the slides.

Interestingly, the hospital made several phone calls to our office demanding the slides be returned to them, even though my understanding – although I am not an attorney - is that legally they are Sarah's property. Therefore, if Sarah ever wishes to prosecute the hospital for misrepresenting the slides, Exhibit A has been stored in a safe place by a third party. How unfortunate that one must take so many precautions because of the dishonesty in hospitals. As of this writing, the hospital has still not accepted our answer, and is still demanding all of the slides. This is even though the slides legally belong to the patient, and her insurance paid the hospital for them.

But of course, such level of corruption should not be surprising, and given my experience with them, is to be expected. Hospitals are required to help anybody stumbling into their emergency departments. This service is an enormous revenue loss, and as the hospitals bleed money out their emergency room doors, there is another sector of the hospital that is the big rainmaker: Oncology. One chemotherapy treatment can be charged to a patient's insurer for up to $50,000 or even $100,000. A cancer patient is worth $180,000 or more to a hospital or cancer clinic. The National Institutes of Health estimate the cost for the first 2 years of breast cancer treatment is $159,442 and $182,655 for Stages III and IV respectively.[22] This is where the hospitals get their largest source of revenue, and this, as you might expect, is why you hear such relentless and aggressive advertising for chemotherapy treatments on the radio.

So is it the timid patient who is more inclined to get cancer? One might think that cancer then offers some protection from a psychic wound, or is like a pearl built by an oyster around an irritating grain of sand. If the cancer patient were so submissive and suppressed that he or she had not expressed himself or herself adequately or cathartically in the past, then maybe that psychic pain needed to be expressed, even if the only alternative, the only feasible means of expression, was to grow a tumor. If one is unable to rebel against one's oppressor, self-inflicted wounds may be the only cathartic release available to the desperate sufferer.

In fact, because passivity seemed to be such a co-morbidity with cancer, I had imagined that it was something that I should also treat, along with the cancer. The way that I did that was, as a typically assertive person myself, to sit back, speak quietly and seldom, assure the cancer patient that he or she was in the driver's seat, and basically try to ease them into a dominant role in the conversation, hoping that it would help to liberate them and allow them to try on a role other than the passive / obedient one for size.

That is, the passivity of cancer patients was just that predictable. Perhaps one out of eight would be assertive, and the rest passive. When almost every cancer patient seems to be less assertive than their family members, the observer begins to think that this cannot be coincidence, that there is something timid or passive about cancer patients in general, as if it were a predictable personality trait, or that passivity itself predisposed a person to have cancer. Or perhaps their pain and pathology made them too glum to talk much.

But as I said earlier, I no longer think that.

Because chemotherapy brings in enough money to turn the heads of the corruptible, I now think that a more likely scenario is this: Patients who give the appearance of being obedient are easier marks for enterprising oncologists. After all, when a doctor has a business to run, it is a lot easier for the doctor to hear, "Yes, Doctor, I'll do as you say," rather than to hear, "You want me to take what kind of poison, doc? Are you out of your mind?" Chemotherapy may be a bit harder to sell to the more assertive members of the population. And those of us who know better than to have any of it would be more of a headache for an oncologist to deal with than an obedient patient, a submissive patient who is inclined to say, "Yes, doctor." So perhaps chemotherapy finds its target market in the more submissive souls among us.

I once had an oncologist call me saying, "This woman must begin chemotherapy right now! She has to start tomorrow." The patient had Stage 1 breast cancer, DCIS, just diagnosed less than a week before. Whose urgency was at work? The patient's? Not so likely as that of the doctor.

I am not alleging any more of a conspiracy theory than would be warranted regarding any other marketing strategy. Ads tailored to your demographic come up on your web browser for similar reasons. Candy is sold in brightly colored packages at kids' eye levels for similar reasons. Halloween costumes are marketed more in October than March for similar reasons, and the reason, as everybody knows is this: Marketing is most effective when its targeted, and if you want to get away with making a lot of money by legally poisoning a person, you'll have an easier time of it with an obedient person rather than a short-tempered, or outspoken, or outside-the-box or in-your-face type person.

And, in my opinion, that is likely why we keep seeing the submissive one of a couple having the cancer diagnosis.

There is one other cancer type, as predictable and easily identified when you meet them as the submissive type. And that is the Pessimist. The Pessimist shows up at our office telling us that they have a terminal cancer, which has us thinking Uh-oh, we're going to have a challenge here. Then often we find out from imaging or pathology that there is a small or easily resected or already resected tumor burden. But more characteristically, we see the scenario described below.

Blood labs are notoriously unreliable with regard to cancer. Imaging can be contradictory or ambiguous. Physical exam has severe limitations, but we do these anyway, on initial consult and then periodically, for further data and information. Thus, over time, we acquire accumulating data points and evidence of which course the disease takes, as the patient's file thickens.

You will recognize the Pessimist by this behavior: The news comes in, arriving in this order: good, ambiguous, good, good, bad, excellent, good, good, and ambiguous. And the Pessimist says, "Aha, bad!" sometimes almost sounding relieved or satisfied. Working with this kind of patient as their health improves can be awkward, because their improving prognosis almost seems disorienting to them, as if they had made some comfort or acceptance or even end-of-life plans with their disease, and now things have to be thought through all over again.

So then if the Passive Type does not necessarily have an active case of cancer, and the Pessimist does not necessarily have an active case of cancer, how much cancer is really out there in the population? Didn't you ever think it odd – and we all know people who have said this – "Thank goodness they did that CT of my abdomen after the car accident, because that's when they found the cancer! And the doctor said if it hadn't been found right then it might've killed me in a few months!" Didn't you ever think it odd that we hear that kind of story so often? At least I hear it from every few new patients. Doesn't it seem a bit statistically improbable that imaging just happened to catch the cancer just in the nick of time to save the patient with chemotherapy?

Might this just have something to do with a story told to me a long time ago by an Emergency Room nurse:

She said when the hospital beds are all full and the waiting room chairs are overflowing, you could be openly bleeding on the floor, and you'll be told, "You'll be fine; you can take care of that at home." Yet when the hospital is empty, "the census is down," as they say, and if you have the misfortune to walk into the ER with a sniffle, it turns out it's the worst thing they've ever seen, and you need a complete workup and to possibly be admitted. If cancer / chemotherapy / radiation are the most lucrative aspect to hospital finances, then are you more likely to be "found" to have cancer when their census is down than on a busy day?

This of course begs the question: If certain patients are singled out to receive the cancer diagnosis because they are more receptive to it, then did those people really have cancer at all?

My question is: Who is auditing the pathologists? The hospital described above that Sarah went to was very eager to have their slides back, slides that their pathologist alleged to demonstrate cancer, but which on careful examination showed no cancer at all to us. They called about once every two weeks for a few months to demand the slides back, that were not their

49

property, from a patient who had not been there since months earlier. We thoroughly examined this patient's slides, because of what had happened with her and the hospital, and we found no cancer. So therefore, is it possible that the massive amount of money that has been flowing through the chemotherapy industry has found its way also to the pathologists? After all, if a pathologist says: clean as a whistle, no cancer here, that is potentially up to a few hundred thousand dollars lost to the institution. And if that same pathologist looks at those same slides of patient tissue and pronounces the presence of cancer, there is all that much more income to be had. Are we so trusting to say that no pressure is ever exerted, no bribe has ever been placed before the pathologist? Is such a suspicion only the subject of fiction? The Fugitive was a film with Harrison Ford, which contained the idea of switching normal and abnormal pathology reports, expressed in a fictional context.[23]

Pathologist Laura Spruill, MD, PhD, of University of South Carolina has acknowledged overdiagnosis of cancer in histopathology labs, and points out very similar appearances of cancerous and non-cancerous tissue, which is commonly deemed cancerous by default.[24]

Certainly, there are people who have cancer, many of them. We find individuals who came in with hard palpable lumps in the breast, bleeding tumors in the colon, massive lumps bulging out the liver, prostate cancer metastasized to the lumbar vertebrae or huge, hard lymph nodes, to name a few types. The pathologist's role here not only confirms what is overwhelmingly likely to be malignancy, but the pathologist lets us have more and more helpful information, especially regarding likely origin of the biopsied tumor.

Another series of incidents that has made me more cynical over time is the eagerness I've seen in oncologists to exploit the pessimism of their patients. Many patients have come to me saying, "It's a good thing I had all that imaging! My tumor wasn't seen on ultrasound or MRI or . . ." Finally, it was this other procedure that found it."

Well, my response to that is that photographs do not lie. If neither the ultrasound nor MRI found your tumor, I would be more inclined to question the existence of that tumor than if it had shown up on such imaging. Certainly, it is theoretically possible for a tumor to escape imaging, but with the sophistication of contemporary imaging technology, this is less likely all the time. If you keep going back for imaging, repeatedly, and of numerous body parts, I think your risk of having something "discovered" increases all the time. If you consider that our ancestors did not have anywhere near the amount of imaging that our current generations indulge in, it seems very likely that they had lumps and bumps all over that nobody had imaged, and that they lived with and likely died with when succumbing to another cause of death. Autopsies often turn up such incidental and benign hematomas, fibroids, adenomas, cysts and such.

Whereas the pessimistic patient assumes that the most pessimistic imaging must be the true one, invalidating other reports, I take all of that imaging as important data points in trying to find out what is really going on with that patient's cancer, especially as it is repeated over time. This is because time, long periods of time, tell the most truth. I may be uncertain today of the tumor burden of the patient in front of me. But five years from now we will be able to look back fairly certain of what this year's situation really is.

And, having been trained in cynicism by repeated strange occurrences in the conventional medical world, I assume nothing. Rather, I look for a preponderance of evidence in order to determine what is happening with a cancer patient. Some of that evidence is what we observe of the money trail and where it may lead. Cancer is such massive business, shouldering the work of keeping hospitals – the nexi of one of the largest growth industries in the US – in the black. It would be naïve to assume that all decisions made with regard to cancer were simply independent of that money, and only related to the best interests of the patient.

Therefore, esteemed readers, just to keep things as honest as possible, let us, you and I, take responsibility for keeping a vigilant eye on such a financially robust industry, just to make sure that our acquaintances, our loved ones, our patients, who are suffering a cancer diagnosis, from possibly a real cancer or perhaps an alleged cancer, are not deceived or otherwise victimized by those with pecuniary priorities.

Chapter 5

Introduction to overwhelming data in Chapters 6, 7 and 8: Some frequently asked questions (FAQs)

Who are you, and what do you do?

I am Colleen Huber, NMD, a Naturopathic Medical Doctor, a licensed physician in Arizona. In my case, I completed the Fellowship of the Naturopathic Oncology Research Institute (FNORI), and so my work is with cancer patients, for the most part.

My clinic, Nature Works Best, is of licensed Naturopathic Medical Doctors (NMDs) at the same address in Tempe, Arizona, USA, for the 11 years of our existence. As of 2017, we are:

- Featured in the documentary Cancer Can Be Killed

- Featured in <u>America's Best Cancer Doctors</u>
  https://www.amazon.com/Americas-Cancer-Doctors-Their-Secrets/dp/1495116530/ref=sr_1_1?ie=UTF8&qid=1492039485&sr=8-1&keywords=america%27s+best+cancer+doctors+and+their+secrets

- Featured in <u>Defeating Cancer</u>:
- https://www.amazon.com/Defeat-Cancer-Integrative-Naturopathic-Medicine/dp/0982513828/ref=sr_1_1?ie=UTF8&qid=1492039515&sr=8-1&keywords=defeating+cance

- A+ rating at BBB (Better Business Bureau)
  https://www.bbb.org/phoenix/business-reviews/naturopaths/nature-works-best-cancer-clinic-in-tempe-az-1000009225

Our goal is to make sure that the cancer patient gets stronger, while we fight the cancer at the cellular and molecular level, until that patient arrives at remission with:

- Evidence of absence of tumor burden, and

- Vitality and strength restored, at least equal to the condition of before the cancer diagnosis.

Our goal is for this to happen with every patient, but many patients must stop the treatments earlier, because insurance coverage is still underperforming for the natural treatments for cancer. Other patients, many others, arrive to our clinic later than optimal timing, after cancer has already spread relentlessly through their bodies. Nevertheless, we do not reject patients for being too sick, and we try our best for all who come to us.

How do you treat cancer?

We are licensed as Naturopathic Medical Doctors and primary care physicians. We use natural treatments only for cancer and other diseases. That is, we use no chemotherapy, radiation or surgery. However, if a patient requests it, we do work with surgeons and oncologists, the formal name for doctors who are cancer specialists. And they work with the mainstream treatments, as well as imaging and labs showing what happens with tumors over time.

If a patient prefers to work only with us, that is okay too. We can order all imaging and labwork. All of that is usually covered by insurance, or at least would apply toward the patient's deductible in many cases. Medicare is an exception, because Medicare does not yet recognize naturopathic medicine.

Do you work with medical doctors?   Does any entity oversee your work?

There are medical doctors who have referred patients to us, and there are medical doctors to whom we have referred patients, based on need.   Medical doctors neither supervise us, nor take direction from us, because we are an independent clinic of Naturopathic

Medical Doctors (NMDs). The government agency that oversees licensed naturopathic physicians is the Naturopathic Medical Board of the state in which those physicians are licensed. In the case of our clinic, that governing body is the Arizona Naturopathic Medical Board.[25]

Our work is also overseen by the Investigational Review Board (IRB) of the American Naturopathic Research Institute / Naturopathic Oncology Research Institute. IRBs were established to protect the rights of human patients. These were established in accordance with the International Declaration of Human Rights: http://www.un.org/en/universal-declaration-human-rights/ and in order to avoid the worst kind of horrors of human experimentation that had been perpetrated throughout the worst periods of human history, IRBs were established in the US – teams of peer clinical researchers as well as at least one non-clinician – as established by the law https://www.hhs.gov/ohrp/regulations-and-policy/regulations/45-cfr-46/index.html - that would evaluate the use of medical treatments or procedures with human beings, according to the specifications of the federal code.

Unfortunately, the prohibition against forced medical treatments is widely ignored in the US medical community, as cancer patients are told every day that they must have chemotherapy, whether they want it or not. For many cancer patients, nobody informs them that there are much safer alternatives to that in natural medicine.

The IRB overseeing our work has submitted our data-gathering from our patients to the Food and Drug

Administration (FDA) and to the Office of Human Research Protections (OHRP), both of which have granted approval, including all previous years in which we applied, and up to the present.

Do you work with oncologists?

There are 2 types of oncologists in our experience: the old-fashioned kind, those who only know about chemotherapy and radiation and surgery, and who are not interested in natural treatments for cancer. Some have shown a lot of hostility toward natural treatments. They have not been very cooperative with us regarding the patients that we share. And this has been detrimental to the patients' wellbeing, because necessary information such as PET scans, MRI's etc. have been delayed and withheld by them.

However, there is a new forward-thinking, well-informed and open-minded type of oncologist, and they are taking an interest in the tumor regression and remission that we have experienced with natural treatments. These oncologists have been helpful and cooperative about sharing information from CT scans, PET scans, blood work, etc., and the patient benefits from this shared information. Fortunately, some of our patients have these newer kinds of oncologists. One such oncologist even told one of our patients that he would do what the patient is doing - that is, the natural treatments - if he himself had cancer, and that he had nothing better to offer for this patient's particular cancer. Another specifically recommended our treatments to another patient as the only therapy. Three other oncologists specifically instructed the patients to continue our natural therapies. That kind of honesty is very welcome to the patient, as well as to the public. Certainly, oncologists can offer some help to some patients. But when they cannot help, it makes most sense for them to welcome other treatments that can make a difference. There is a genuine desire on the part of many mainstream doctors to act with the patient's best interests as a priority, regardless of where that road may go.

If a patient wants to consult with an oncologist who will be open-minded to the natural treatments that the patient chooses, we can refer to any of a number of different oncologists if the patient requests the referral.

Why don't you advertise on billboards and the radio, like Mayo and others?

MD Anderson, Cancer Treatment Centers of America, Mayo and other cancer conglomerates seem to be advertising everywhere. You can hardly turn on a radio or TV without an ad from a cancer hospital. Their billboards are all over our most congested highways. Their soundbites are everywhere.

Soundbites may work well enough to advertise for chemotherapy, because everybody has an idea of what it is. However, natural treatments for cancer are still unfamiliar to much of the American public, and require more of an introduction than simply a commercial. This is why we explain on our website what we do and the results that we have had, while preserving patient anonymity.

What natural treatments do you use?

It's important to understand that that depends entirely on the patient. Each of our cancer patients came in with a different type of cancer and even different metastases.

As for an example of a specific treatment, let's say a cancer patient has lung involvement. Then we will deliver natural treatments to the lungs by way of a nebulizer. This has been helpful with both primary lung cancers as well as secondary metastases to the lungs. What we put in there is a combination of herbs and nutrients, in a form that is tolerable to the airways, and with specific attention to the patients' needs.

We also offer intravenous anti-cancer nutrients, such as high doses of Vitamin C and other anti-cancer nutrients that benefit normal cells while killing cancer cells.

Linus Pauling is the only person in history to be awarded two solo Nobel prizes. His work with Vitamin C and cancer was groundbreaking decades ago. Now we know that we can use much higher doses of Vitamin C than at that time without side effects, when we use it intravenously, and get even better results than previously.

Certain herbs have shown a tremendous effect in slowing the growth of cancer or shrinking tumors and inhibiting metastases, so we use those when appropriate. Renée Caisse was a Canadian nurse who worked with the Ojibwa people, and together they put together a formula of herbs that has shown good results for many patients, called Essiac, so we often use that, but I prefer not to use those herbs alone.

Several other cancer-fighting strategies are available from nature. Cancer creates an acid environment, and seems to adapt to it, which I will discuss later on. Therefore, we incorporate alkaline treatments, because most types of cancer cells seem to thrive in acidity.

Dr. Tullio Simoncini is well known for his work with sodium bicarbonate and cancer. He sees cancer as closely related to fungal conditions, which are intolerant of an alkaline environment. So he uses sodium bicarbonate by injection. Although Dr. Simoncini has done groundbreaking work, this is one piece of a very large and complex puzzle. We do need the other treatments as well to be really effective. Several other natural substances will also provide helpful alkalinity. We use some intravenously, and some are taken orally. The ones we like best are the ones that are attracted to the tumors and more active there, with least disturbance to other cells.

The different treatments for different patients can be expensive for some patients, which then further limits the number of treatments that they opt to receive.

How successful have you been?

Chapter 7 gives detailed data of the results that we have had with cancer treatment. Of those going into remission, it has taken an average of 3.7 months from when we first met with them to confirmation of total remission (no tumor load left in the body, or in the case of lymphoma or leukemia, normal labs). Very few patients whom we have gotten into remission have had a recurrence of their cancer, except for those who disagreed with our main dietary recommendation, and another who had undiscovered metastases prior to treatment, which in her case had been too short, and others for whom current imaging and other findings are ambiguous.

How do you handle safety at your clinic?

Safety at our clinic, and in natural medicine generally, is far easier to achieve than with chemotherapy. At our clinic, we have given over 31,000 IV nutrient treatments, and we have never had to call 911 for a patient receiving an IV. The close attention of our doctors, registered nurses and medical assistants to the patients has ensured that they do well and that they are tolerating our treatments. Patients who have sensitivity or intolerance to one or another component of the treatment, which is a relatively unusual occurrence, discontinue that part of the treatment. This is still generally successful, because there are a number of safe and effective ways to fight cancer from nature.

Does insurance cover any of this?

Things are changing very rapidly here. Recently, the major insurance companies have begun to cover naturopathic treatments more than before, as they realize that we save them quite a bit of money over mainstream medicine. Unfortunately, Medicare and Medicaid are still not covering natural treatments.

United Health Care, Health Net and Humana have

been somewhat better at covering naturopathic medicine. Others are starting to catch up. Even Blue Cross/Blue Shield, which never used to cover naturopathic services are beginning to bring themselves up to date. The most common objection of the insurance companies to the natural treatments is that they are "experimental." However, many of these treatments have had a better history of sustained remission from cancer than a lot of the chemotherapy drugs.

We submit our bills to insurance. Although payment is due for each treatment at the time of service, we try to get a patient's insurance company to reimburse by submitting the proper codes for diagnosis and treatment.

Does the FDA approve of any of this?

The scope of practice for a Naturopathic Medical Doctor in the State of Arizona as well as a number of other licensed states includes the following: primary care practice (office consults, physical exams, laboratory tests and imaging), natural medicine (nutrition, IV nutrients, herbs, acupuncture, homeopathy, physical medicine, hydrotherapy) as well as some of mainstream medicine (minor surgery, prescription of pharmaceuticals if indicated).

For cancer, all treatments that we use are natural unpatented substances, and all are available in some form or other to the general public, over the counter. However, the quantities and form differ greatly, if you really want to have a fighting chance against such a vicious disease as cancer. Some of this has to be given intravenously in order to be really effective against cancer. You can't just get enough or the right amounts and proportion and form of these simply by taking them orally. Although for certain items, we ask all of our patients, whether they have cancer or not, to go buy this or that item at the health food stores. So we located our office near a number of health food stores.

So yes, it's all legal, all within the scope of practice of naturopathic physicians here in Arizona, licensed by the State of Arizona, with oversight by the Naturopathic Physicians Board of Medical Examiners, and our medical schools are accredited by the US Department of Education. At this writing, there are 20 states and 3 additional US jurisdictions that license naturopathic medicine. They are:

- Alaska
- Arizona
- California
- Colorado
- Connecticut
- Hawaii
- Kansas
- Maine
- Maryland
- Massachusetts
- Minnesota
- Montana
- New Hampshire
- North Dakota
- Oregon
- Pennsylvania
- Rhode Island
- Utah
- Vermont
- Washington
- Washington, DC
- Puerto Rico
- Virgin Islands

What happens to the patients?

First, they start feeling better and their energy comes back. The vitality of the patients usually begins within several weeks after we start treating them, long before we have evidence from ultrasound or CT scans, MRI or PET scans of tumors turning necrotic, or shrinking tumors, or tumors turning to inactive tissue. We look for evidence coming back of shrinking tumors or tumors that are no longer there.

There are also many patients who do not have successful results. The more damage that cancer has caused to the body and the more widespread metastases prior to diagnosis, the harder it is to defeat.

Every year, we survey patients to determine ongoing remission or recurrence, and various parameters of health, such as frequency of exercise and dietary choices.

Profiles of some of our patients

The following dozen cases are listed in no particular order, but are a representative sample of the experiences of our patients.

Case 1:

A woman with endometrial cancer came in with a tumor the size of a grapefruit, with such a deadly form of this particular cancer that there are no survivors of it in the medical literature except for this patient. Neither chemotherapy, nor radiation nor surgery could eliminate it. It grew back each time. The tumor was eliminated in 2008 with our treatments, and the patient has kept her very active career ever since. There is still no evidence of any recurrence.

Case 2:

A woman in her fifties had malignant melanoma, which is one of the most dangerous kinds of cancers and the most dangerous of the skin cancers. By the time we met her, it had already metastasized to her brain. This patient chose a combination of surgery, radiation and our natural cancer-fighting treatments, which we continued until she went into remission and continued an active life with recreational travel.

Case 3:

A man in his fifties had prostate cancer and chose only our natural treatments in 2008. He did not want to have any of the mainstream treatments. After less than three months of natural treatments, he is still in remission. He continues to ride his bicycle several miles a day and worked two strenuous jobs and now one strenuous full-time job.

Case 4:

This is a patient who eventually died of cancer. It was inoperable pancreatic cancer, and the two tumors had actually shrunk considerably, with one disappearing completely, during the course of our natural treatments alone. This patient enjoyed a high quality of health, very active physically and feeling good during the first few months of our natural treatments. However, as things started to look very good, there arose different viewpoints about the best way to proceed throughout the healing process, particularly dietary choices, and the initial success turned to very aggressive metastases throughout the body. We can help patients avoid this outcome.

Case 5:

A man in his fifties with colon cancer chose a combination of surgery, chemotherapy and our natural treatments. Among all these interventions, the patient experienced a reduction in his cancer of 80% from chemotherapy and natural treatments alone, beginning after the initial surgery. However, at the same time, complications from his surgery took him back into the hospital with a very high morphine dose, and without recovery. We can help discuss the risk of adhesions with your surgeon prior to surgery, to help avoid this excruciatingly painful adverse result of certain surgeries.

Case 6:

A woman in her fifties with breast cancer is considering all options and for right now just receiving our natural treatments and remains stable and well with a high quality of life and activity.

Case 7:

A woman in her seventies with breast cancer also considered all her options and decided to just receive our natural treatments. She is now in remission with a high quality of life and wellbeing.

Case 8:

A woman in her forties with breast cancer chose lumpectomy and our natural treatments. She is now in remission, and she has resumed an active life with recreational travel.

Case 9:

A man in his seventies has lung cancer, which has now reduced in volume more than 90% with a combination of radio ablation and our natural treatments.

Case 10:

A man in his seventies with leukemia has been through chemotherapy and a number of natural treatments. After treating him for some months, his numbers remain stable. Although not yet in remission, this man's quality of life remains quite high. He is very physically active, and rides his bicycle several miles a day and helped a friend build a cabin with their own hands.

Case 11:

This patient in her forties has had primary colon cancer, primary ovarian cancer and primary uterine cancer. When she came to us after surgery, there were metastases as well, and her condition was weak, fatigued and delicate. With only our natural treatments, the metastases disappeared and the patient's improved vitality and new robust energy was quite dramatic. Her travel schedule is active. She is still in remission over seven years later.

Case 12:

A man in his forties with Non-Hodgkins lymphoma came to us for natural cancer treatment. He had already been through chemotherapy. With the natural treatments that we have used, he maintained a high quality of living, active in his work and hiking in the local mountains. He went into remission while continuing the natural treatments alone. Then we did not hear from him for several years. Then he came back with a widely-metastasized cancer, having resumed chemotherapy. This time, we were not so fortunate as to be able to help him. We can help advise future patients how to avoid this outcome.

Chapter 6

**Risks and benefits of chemotherapy vs.
Risks and benefits of natural cancer treatments**

**If we look at the two shaded columns on the right side of Table B, chemotherapy was far more correlated with death,
and not having chemotherapy was far more correlated with remission.**

Our clinic studied the results of treatment of all 379 consecutive cancer patients, all types of cancer, all stages, without exception, who came to our clinic over the course of 8 years and stayed at least two weeks in our care. We opened our clinic in 2006, and began to collect data from the patients who came to us. We stopped collecting data in 2014 due to the cumbersome nature of trying to reach a quickly increasing number of people. Patients did not necessarily continue with the same doctor as we grew, which impaired continuity of care. Also, voice mail and competition with enormous amounts of spam e-mail further hindered efforts at ongoing contact with patients who had left our clinic years earlier. So we stopped looking at this particular information in 2014.

However, every year we now survey patients while they are at our clinic, and ask more limited and more focused questions than we used to, every year focusing on a somewhat different topic. In 2015, we asked questions regarding a long list of foods and beverages. In 2016, we asked questions regarding outlook: optimism vs pessimism. Most years we ask questions regarding nutrition and exercise.

This article addresses specifically the difference in outcome between those patients that had chemotherapy and those who did not, among those who chose to come to our clinic and had natural treatments for cancer. Of course, those who did not come to our clinic did not have information that was available to us for our study. So all of the following patients had natural treatments for their cancers, and are therefore not representative of the whole of US cancer patients. Let's compare those who had chemotherapy with those who did not.

Summarized outcomes of naturopathic treatment of 379 consecutive cancer patients
Table A

	Outcome	Number of patients	Average number of months this group of patients stayed for treatments *	Number in each group also receiving chemotherapy	Number in each group also receiving radiation	Number in each group also receiving surgery
a	Remission or assumed remission	175	3.7	12	11	59
b	Still being treated, not yet in remission	22	4.0	1	0	3
c	Died while still only in our care, following all of our protocols	32	2.2	0	1	1
d	Iatrogenic death in hospitals, conventional medicine	22	2.7	15	4	7
e	Of those who left early, number who died after leaving (except for DDD)**	45	2.7	2	3	10
f	Death after dietary dispute	12	No data	1	1	3
g	No current information but never known to be in remission	46	1.4	5	1	10
h	Remission occurred elsewhere	8	No data	4	1	0
i	Waiting to know status, or conflicting information	17	No data	5	2	6
	Total	379		45	24	99

*This column has not been updated since 2010, due to the labor-intensive nature of this research, and not much expected change or significance of any change.
** Please see legend of abbreviations at the head of Table 1. For example, DDD: death after dietary dispute.

Now let's summarize the above table to look at all of those in remission, and whether they had chemotherapy or not:

Table B

	Number of patients	Number also receiving chemo-therapy	Number not receiving chemo-therapy	Ratio of those not having chemo-therapy to total	% of total not having chemo-therapy	% of total having chemo-therapy
Remission or assumed remission	175	12	163	163/175	93%	7%
Iatrogenic death in hospitals, conven-tional medicine	22	15	7	7/22	32%	68%
All patients	379	45	334	334/379	88%	12%

We see in Table B that 88% of all the patients we treated did not have chemotherapy. However, 93% of those patients in remission did not have chemotherapy. Therefore, remission was more highly correlated with not having chemotherapy treatment than in the average patient. However, it is even more likely that chemotherapy was not helpful, or was harmful to cancer patients generally for this reason: People who choose to have naturopathic treatment for cancer are probably the least likely people to have chosen to have chemotherapy treatment. So therefore, the 88% figure is artificially high, and again not representative of the US cancer population as a whole.

The cornerstone of conventional treatment of cancer patients in the United States and many other countries is chemotherapy treatment. Of those who attended our clinic, and who later died in hospitals or conventional medicine clinics, only 32% did not have chemotherapy. 68% (=15 of 22) of those dying in conventional medical settings had received chemotherapy treatment.

If we look at the two shaded columns on the right side of Table B, chemotherapy was more likely to result in death, and not having chemotherapy was far more likely to result in remission.

Let's look more specifically at what happened to the patients who left to have chemotherapy:

Table C:
Results for patients who left our treatments in order to have chemotherapy prior to 2013

Went into remission following chemo-therapy	Died following chemotherapy	Not in remission, but surviving both chemotherapy and cancer as of mid-2013	Evidence of remission from our treatments alone prior to starting chemotherapy	Total who left our clinic to have chemotherapy (total of all outcomes)
4	9	5	6	24

This table has not been updated since July 2013. It shows that leaving our treatments to pursue

73

chemotherapy only possibly benefited 4 of the 24 patients who had left (17%), but 9 others died after leaving for chemotherapy (38%). However, it is possible that those 4 would have gone into remission if they had continued with our treatments alone. This table has not been updated since 2013, because others who were thought to have left for chemotherapy could not be reached by phone. As of now, we have not attributed either pessimistic or optimistic outcomes to those we cannot reach; we simply record "NFI" for "no further information" in Table 1 of our long paper.[26] Sometimes good or bad information comes much later. In 2014, we were absolutely delighted to welcome to our clinic visits from two cancer survivors, after only our treatments, who had not been in contact with us for 5 years and 4 years respectively (Patients #288 and 295 of Table 1). One lives in an RV trailer, and happened to be passing through our area again. Similar long absences have ended in unexpected and very pleasant visits in each year since.

Of the patients who left our treatments to pursue chemotherapy, comparing only those who then went into remission or died, (13 total), 4 went into remission and 9 died. This is a 31% short-term success rate for chemotherapy, and a 69% fatality rate for chemotherapy among those who left to pursue it. This is similar to the figure of 68% in Table B, for those who died in hospitals at some point in time after having chemotherapy treatments.

Chemotherapy is known to be toxic, life-threatening and at times fatal. It is known to have a very poor track record long-term.[27]

It is a long-held (and heavily purchased) dogmatic belief that chemotherapy is the weapon of choice against cancer. There are some problems with this:

One, there usually is no choice given. Newly diagnosed cancer patients are not told that there are any options other than chemotherapy. If a patient suggests to the oncologist that alternatives exist, that patient is usually told: But your cancer would respond especially well to chemotherapy; therefore, that is the treatment that you should have.

Two, chemotherapy has been oversold for its anti-cancer effect, and has been falsely promoted as effective against all cancers. A July 2017 article in Science Translational Medicine [28] found that chemotherapy actually *increases* the risk of metastasis. This progression to metastasis is what makes cancer especially deadly and beyond medical control.

Although chemotherapy generally dramatically reduces the size of tumors, not only does the remaining cancer metastasize more readily, but it also becomes more resilient to subsequent treatment.

After 10 years of working with cancer patients, I have become more and more convinced that the worst thing a cancer patient can do is choose to have chemotherapy. Those are the people who get sick and die, in my experience. Whereas those who avoid it have generally had much better success[29] in eliminating cancer from their bodies for the long-term.

Chemotherapy has been a financial boon to hospitals. Whereas "health" insurance has been slow or stubborn about paying for cheaper alternatives, those same insurance companies lavish enormous sums on oncology clinics for exorbitantly priced chemotherapy drugs, some of which can cost tens of thousands of dollars per dose.

The chemotherapy paradigm has been a misguided paradigm for cancer treatment, ever since it was first recycled from World War I and II chemical weapons. Isn't it time to consider the many safe and effective natural alternatives [30] that exist?

The above information should give people pause before choosing to embark on chemotherapy.

Chapter 7

Defeating cancer requires more than one treatment method:
A 10-year retrospective case series using multiple nutritional and herbal agents, 2016 update

© Colleen Huber, NMD

There has been no financial support for this research. The author has received no funding, nor is affiliated with any industrial or commercial entity other than her own private medical practice.

December 30, 2016. This paper is an update of the 2009, 2010, 2011, 2012, 2013, 2014 and 2015 editions of this paper.

Abstract

INTRODUCTION: Research has shown that for cancer to occur in the body multiple normal functions must break down. Therefore multiple-component treatments may be the only successful way to treat cancer. We used well-tolerated natural substances to assess their usefulness in combination cancer-disrupting therapy.[*] The following has been the goal of our clinic in treating cancer patients: It is not enough to repair genetic damage or to stop angiogenesis and neglect to reverse all other cancer-causing problems. It is also not enough to attack metastases and leave the primary tumor in a comfortable environment. In order to defeat cancer, it must be attacked at every level and with every method necessary to reverse cancer's multiple-layered assault on the body, even if that means that some of the various treatments have redundant effects. And this all must be accomplished while maintaining the maximum possible wellbeing of the patient, and without sickening or weakening the patient. This has been the mission of our clinic.

---

[*] Anti-neoplastic is an inaccurate term to describe the effects of natural substances with anti-cancer effect. Conventional chemotherapy is anti-neoplastic in that it interferes with either DNA and RNA function (alkylating agents, topoisomerase inhibitors) or DNA and RNA synthesis (anti-metabolites) or other aspects of cell reproduction (anti-microtubule agents). In either case, cells are unable to reproduce, so that new cells are damaged first, and we see the results in lost hair (most obviously), an excoriated GI tract and arrested tumor growth. The natural anti-cancer treatments on the other hand do not target new growth indiscriminately (cancer, embryo, hair, GI lining), but rather target the 7 major mechanisms of cancer reproduction and growth described below. Hence, throughout this paper, we call them "cancer-disrupting" substances.

METHODS: We treated a total of 379 patients with cancer from October 2006, when we opened our practice, until July 1, 2014, when we stopped collecting data for the 2014 update of this paper, originally written in 2009. Data from all 379 patients who came to us with a diagnosis of cancer up to that time are included in this paper, excluding only those cancer patients who decided against further treatment after less than two weeks in our care. Patients' stage is recorded as the stage at first arrival to our clinic, which is not necessarily the stage when first diagnosed. We treated with natural methods alone, choosing among methods with research-established cancer-disrupting effect, both oral and intravenous, dietary and supplemented, nutritional and herbal, having a preference for those with high patient tolerance and compatibility, and varying with individual needs and tolerance, according to the standard naturopathic principle of "Treat the whole person."

FINDINGS: Many patients voluntarily left our practice, against our advice, primarily for financial reasons, while still having cancer. Of the remaining patients, 175 either went into confirmed, complete remission, which we define by no evidence of cancer remaining in the body on imaging, or have remained in good to excellent wellbeing, as determined retrospectively by prolonged stable health of at least 6 months after leaving our care and needing no other physician supervised cancer care, and as confirmed by annual telephone conversation with either the patient or a family member. Those patients in remission stayed in our care an average of 3.7 months; those who left, 2.7 months, (this data last measured in 2010). Eight additional patients went into remission after leaving our clinic, and while being treated at a different clinic, and it is unlikely that our treatments were the decisive factor in that remission. We were still treating 22 patients at July 1, 2014 plus giving ongoing maintenance treatments to some of those who are still in remission. 44 died while still our patients. Of those 44, 12 died after a significant dietary dispute with us. That is 32 patients died although they received our treatments and complied with our requested diet. 22 more were killed by hospital procedures and/or chemotherapy and/or radiation side effects while still our patients. 45 total patients chose to have chemotherapy while having our treatments. Yet, of the 175 who went into remission, only 12 had chosen to have chemotherapy while having our treatments. Stages 1, 2, 3 and early Stage 4 patients at start of treatment had much better outcomes than late Stage 4 patients in general.

INTERPRETATION: The 32 patients who complied with our dietary and treatment protocol, and still did not survive their cancers must be seen as an 8% failure rate if considered of all 379 patients, or a 15% failure rate if taken of the 210 patients who stayed to complete our treatments. Therefore, these treatment strategies are still not adequate to eliminate all patients' cancers and must be further developed. However, our success rate of 93% in steadfast patients following all protocols as recommended, from Stage I through early Stage IV (Table 5) is unprecedented and unequalled in both conventional and natural medicine in all clinics that report their results in detail as we do in this paper. There is also a 93% rate of sustained remission in individual patients who elect to follow our recommendation to have monthly follow-up treatments. 26 of those 28 patients are still in remission. (Table 9). 27 of those patients are alive and well (97%). Because of this consistent success in treating cancer since 2006, we believe that the experiences of over 300 cancer patients detailed below have demonstrated the need for simultaneous well-tolerated cancer-disrupting treatments, across all cancers and stages of cancer.

Introduction

Cancer treatment has been constrained by the prevailing view that a single agent must be isolated and tested for its either successful or failing role as the therapeutic agent to eliminate cancer. This viewpoint is disastrous for most patients, for the following reasons. Many agents are needed to fight cancer, primarily because it arises after several normal mechanisms break down, and because cancer preys on the body in numerous ways simultaneously, and because no single agent, whether chemotherapeutic or natural, has yet been found that has enough cancer-disrupting strategic effects to reverse all of those abnormalities in all patients, in effect, to be "the cure" for cancer. At our clinic in Tempe, AZ, USA we therefore simultaneously employ multiple naturally derived, unpatented, and therefore inexpensive, substances for use in cancer patients.

Background

As John Boik has described, cancer becomes possible, and has its only opportunity to arise in the body, when seven different events, such as genetic damage, angiogenesis, immune system evasion, etc. all occur,[31] as listed below. Then, once established,

81

cancer is adaptable enough to be able to thrive and grow with the continuation of just one or a few of those unfortunate events.

Boik describes the seven pro-cancer events as follows:

1) genetic instability or vulnerability to mutation, necessarily the first of the variety of events that lead to a tumor;
2) abnormal gene expression, in this case that produce proteins that facilitate cancer, or at least do not prevent it;
3) abnormal and autonomous cell signal transduction, which allows cancer cells to grow through auto-stimulation rather than depending on growth factors from other cells;
4) Abnormal cell-to-cell communication, which sets a tumor apart from its neighboring cells metabolically, leaving the tumor in a position to ignore homeostatic mechanisms and, unlike cells throughout the rest of the body, to act in the best interests of the tumor rather than in the best interests of the host organism.
5) Angiogenesis, the creation of blood vessels and resultant hoarding by the tumor of disproportionately large amounts of blood-borne molecules;
6) Invasion and metastasis, which not only results from the aggressive nature of the tumor, but also the low tensile strength (sometimes from previous injury), and too friable nature of the surrounding normal tissue and basement membranes;
7) Evasion of the immune system, which involves both camouflage functions and immune-disabling functions of cancer cells.

Once established in the body, cancer seems to have the ability to thrive and reproduce despite most of the efforts against it by chemotherapy oncologists, and without necessarily requiring all seven of the above pro-cancer events to still be in place. Therefore, without certain knowledge of the precise mechanisms governing any one patient's cancer, and without the luxury of time to learn of all those mechanisms in each individual patient, any therapy that targets fewer than those seven major disturbances leaves the body of the cancer patient potentially vulnerable to the disastrous result of allowing continued growth of existing tumors. Shortchanging the patient of a diverse range of available, effective, well-tolerated, well-targeted, compatible, complementary and feasible treatment options also would allow too many of the conditions to persist that gave rise to tumors previously and may do so again. This would leave fertile ground and pro-neoplastic conditions that produced the cancer in the first place. For this reason, successful cancer therapy should be multi-purposed and with multiple agents, many more than are now used with each patient by chemotherapy oncologists.

We have used natural therapies for cancer treatment, because they are well adapted for multi-agent use. Unrefined plant materials have tens of thousands or more phytochemical components, originally useful for protecting a plant from extreme or adverse conditions in its environment, and ultimately employed as described below by naturopathic physicians in adaptation to the needs of the human patient. The nutrients, each with a well-established role in the complex tapestry of metabolic pathways, serve to enable defensive functions of the body, such as strengthening, repair and immune activity. Licensed naturopathic physicians, because of thorough medical training, having more classroom hours and more than twice the number of courses in medical school as medical doctors[32] [33], as well as extensive training in the use of natural agents, are well suited to choose appropriate combinations of natural therapies for the individual cancer patient. We also take advantage of the greater compatibility among natural substances than is possible with combinations of numerous pharmaceuticals. It seems obvious that a meal may contain many different foods without the need for conscious consideration of potential interactions among nutrients and plant molecules. In the same way, we have combined many different nutrients and plant materials in each cancer patient's treatment protocol, with regard for the specific cancer burden in the body, the origin of the cancer, the nature of that particular patient's cancer and any co-morbid conditions.

Materials and Methods

Dietary interventions are of the utmost importance in cancer therapy, especially keeping blood sugar low. Otto Warburg, Nobel physicist showed in 1926 that glucose fuels cancer growth and that cancer is dependent on glucose for fermentation as its default metabolism.[34] The significant majority of research on the subject establishes a correlation between blood glucose and tumor growth. Using PET imaging preferentially for tumor evaluation, clinicians make use of the fact that tumors take up blood glucose disproportionately over benign tissue, which implies an especially glucose-dependent metabolism in cancer cells.

Research has shown a correlation between blood sugar or glycemic load and cancer growth for pancreatic cancer,[35] [36] [37] [38] breast cancer,[39] [40] [41] [42] prostate cancer,[43] [44] gastric cancer, [45] [46] colorectal cancer,[47] [48] [49] [50] ovarian cancer,[51] [52] endometrial cancer,[53] [54] and liver and biliary tract cancers.[55] [56] Given all of this evidence, it would be reckless for a physician to allow a cancer patient to assume that sugar intake is harmless. We therefore ask all of our cancer patients to avoid sweeteners, such as sugar, honey, maple syrup, corn syrup, as well as fruit juices, because such foods tend to have the highest glycemic indices. Use of stevia is encouraged if and when a sweetener is desired. For the same reason, we asked patients to also limit other refined carbohydrates, specifically flour products. Whole natural foods: vegetables, fruits, whole grains, eggs, dairy and other animal proteins are encouraged as the entire diet, with the widest available variety in those groups. Many patients arrive to our clinic already consuming all of those types of foods. Some patients have chosen a vegan diet. Others have chosen an ovo-lacto-vegetarian diet. Many others are omnivores. We have not actively pushed our patients to one or the other of these diets, because we tried to maintain the primary dietary focus on the avoidance of sweeteners. Use of soy is discouraged because of its mineral-depleting and phytoestrogenic components, which in some studies has been linked to a possible association with cancer.

Of equal emphasis with diet are the intravenous nutrients that we administer three times per week to each cancer patient. These consist of high-dose intravenous vitamin C (ascorbic acid), as well as other nutrients chosen for specific cancer-disrupting effect with regard to the patient's type of cancer. For solid malignant tumors, we address the problem of pH, by infusing both sodium bicarbonate to alkalinize systemically, as well as other specifically anti-cancer nutrients, tailored to the individual patient's tumor load, type of cancer and other health circumstances. B vitamins and minerals and other nutrients are often added for synergistic effect with Vitamin C, or because of their history of reducing and eliminating tumors, or their usefulness in converting malignant tumors into benign tissue, but primarily for their driving the citric acid cycle, and starving the pyruvate-to-lactate machinery characteristic of cancer. So a major goal is to push the citric acid cycle, and to disrupt the anaerobic glycolysis used by cancer to convert glucose to lactic acid.

Naturopathic training emphasizes the treatment of the individual with regard to the entire symptom picture. Therefore, there is no specific formula to be repeated in a rigid way from one patient to the next, or even for the same patient from one day to the next. Quantities of the different components of this combination vary among individual patients depending on symptoms, signs and type of cancer. Quantities also vary as the patient's needs change. All components are kept far below the LD50 for each component, and are only administered if they have not produced any side effects in our patients.

Research has established that ascorbic acid taken orally cannot attain sufficiently high concentrations in the bloodstream to kill cancer cells.[57][58] However, intravenous use of ascorbic acid has been shown to rise to concentrations that have killed cancer cells in vivo [59 60 61] and in vitro.[62 63 64] The ascorbic acid that we use is in much higher dose than would be tolerated orally, yet at a level where there is sufficient concentration of vitamin C in the bloodstream to create a substantial concentration of the products of vitamin C in the extracellular fluid.[65] Intravenous doses of ascorbic acid have been found to produce from 25 to 70 times as much plasma concentration as may be attained by oral dosing.[66] Research has confirmed that Vitamin C in such high concentration kills cancer cells while leaving normal tissue unharmed.[67] [68] Indeed the cancer patients whom we treat do not have side effects from these treatments, with few exceptions. Three of the exceptions were allergies to specific B vitamins in three individuals. Two of the three went into remission after we had removed the offending agent early on.

In addition to this directly and selectively cytotoxic effect on cancer cells, vitamin C has been shown to form collagen[69] and to inhibit hyaluronidase[70] leading to stronger membrane integrity and tensile strength[71] of normal tissue, which inhibits invasion[72] and thus metastases.

Empirical data shows an inverse correlation between vitamin D intake and cancer incidence.[73] [74] [75] Research over the last decade has confirmed the essential role that Vitamin D plays in cancer prevention and treatment.[76 77 78 79] Vitamin D has been shown to induce differentiation,[80] and apoptosis,[81] to reduce proliferation by effect on signal transduction,[82] to improve intercellular communication by means of gap junction communication preservation,[83] to inhibit angiogenesis,[84 85] and to inhibit metastasis.[86] At our clinic, most cancer patients are prescribed a regular dose of Vitamin D3 that is compatible with customary sunlight exposure, current pharmaceuticals if any, as well as the assessed condition of the liver and gallbladder and calcium metabolizing mechanisms.

Vitamin A is a less-widely appreciated but quite crucial part of the treatment protocol for its immune-stimulating property[87] and inhibition of cancer cell migration[88]. Another very important quality of Vitamin A with regard to neoplastic cells is its ability to introduce differentiation.[89] [90] It has also been shown to induce apoptosis in cancer cells,[91] as well as growth inhibition.[92] Although there have been some objections made to Vitamin A for an allegedly competitive and detrimental effect to vitamin D,[93] vitamin A seems to be vindicated by a preponderance of older research that supports the use of vitamin A and vitamin D dosed together.[94] [95] [96]

We frequently add the recommendation to take Essiac tea (Resperin Canada Limited, Waterloo, Ontario, Canada), because of its long history in North America, over most of the last century of folk use (outside of conventional medicine) against a wide variety of cancers. Essiac was developed by a Canadian nurse, René Caisse, together with the Ojibwe people of Canada. It is a combination of four herbs, Arctium lappa, Rheum palmatum, Rumex acetosella, and Ulmus fulva. Later versions of Essiac, using additional herbs with some pro-estrogenic effect, have been linked to breast tissue proliferation,[97] and we do not recommend those altered formulas. Essiac has been found to have in vitro cytotoxic effects specifically against neoplastic cells, without damage to normal cells.[98] Its main effect seems to be protective against

DNA damage.[99]   It also seems to have anti-proliferative effect.[100]

For different cancers there are additional appropriate treatments. For example, Kenneth Proefrock NMD has done extensive original work with nebulizers, as well as in many other areas of medicine, which he taught us to use with lung cancer patients, as well as others with metastases in the lungs, to good effect.[101] Whereas all of the rest of our treatments arrive to the lungs by way of the bloodstream, Dr. Proefrock has introduced such nebulized botanicals and nutrients as required by the individual patient by way of the airways, thus carrying cancer-disrupting treatments to lung tissue via its other major port of entry.

Findings

The data obtained from our patients in 2015 differs considerably from data obtained over the previous 6 years. The difference was that from 2009 through 2014 we called all surviving patients every summer to ask about their wellbeing. However, in 2015 we mailed a questionnaire to each of our surviving patients. 97 of our cancer survivors mailed back the completed questionnaire in a timely way to prepare a database for presentation at the 2015 Euro Cancer Summit. This is likely more than one quarter of our surviving cancer patients. Most who did not respond told us they had not yet had time to respond to the whole questionnaire. Our paper on cancer survivors' diets discusses the results of this questionnaire in detail.[102]

The data obtained in 2016 involved questions of a psychological nature as well as some questions from earlier years. This also resulted from a mailed questionnaire. Unfortunately, a combination of exhaustive and intrusive questioning, lost or forgotten mail and survey fatigue were the most likely causes of having only 69 responses to our 2016 questionnaires.[103]

Of the 379 cancer patients whom we had treated long-term through the end of June 2014, all came to us with a diagnosis of cancer from another physician, none originally diagnosed by us. Those who are reported below stayed for at least two weeks in our care, which involved intravenous cancer-disrupting nutrients. As of June 30 of each year, we stopped collecting data for that year, and we began annual telephone outreach to all of the surviving patients who have been diagnosed with cancer, and who have stayed at least two weeks in our care. Those results are reported below. Since we began collecting this data for the 2009 edition of this paper, automated telephone dialing seems to have become more pervasive in the United States, and the public's defense against such frequent interruptions have become more varied and creative. Therefore, it is now harder to reach our patients and their families. If a patient was referred by another, sometimes we have to return to the source of the referral for updated information. Of the 379 individual patients meeting the above criteria, 44 have died of cancer while still our patients under our care, and of those 44, 12 did not comply with our main dietary advice to avoid sweeteners. Therefore, 44 − 12 = 32 patients died while under our care and complying with all of our protocols. 175 have gone into complete remission or assumed complete remission, substantiated by PET/CT or other imaging, and/or biopsy, and/or stable good health for at least 6 months after stopping our treatments.

Specific results are shown in Table 1. Table 1 is too large to fit in a print paperback such as this, unless the type is at least 7 point. Smaller type is not feasible for print clarity. Please see the whole of Table 1 at the site www.NatureWorksBest.com, and click on "documented." A summary of Table 1 is shown in Table 2.

Table 1: Outcomes of naturopathic treatment of 379 consecutive cancer patients[104]

The results in Table 1 are summarized as follows:

Table 2: Summarized outcomes of naturopathic treatment of 379 consecutive cancer patients

	Outcome	Number of patients	Average number of months this group of patients stayed for treat-ments *	Number in each group also receiving chemo-therapy	Number in each group also receiving radiation	Number in each group also receiving surgery
a	Remission or assumed remission	175	3.7	12	11	59
b	Still being treated, not yet in remission	22	4.0	1	0	3
c	Died while still only in our care, following all of our protocols	32	2.2	0	1	1
d	Iatrogenic death in	22	2.7	15	4	7

	hospitals or conventional clinics					
e	Of those who left before finishing treatment, number who died after leaving (except for DDD)**	45	2.7	2	3	10
f	Death after dietary dispute	12	No data	1	1	3
g	No current information but never known to be in remission	46	1.4	5	1	10
h	Remission occurred elsewhere	8	No data	4	1	0
i	Waiting to know status, or conflicting information	17	No data	5	2	6
	Total	379		45	24	99

*This column has not been updated since 2010, due to the labor-intensive nature of this research, and not much expected change or significance of any change.
** Please see legend of abbreviations at the head of Table 1. For example, DDD: death after dietary dispute.

I called all of the cancer survivors every summer until 2014 to annually update the data for this paper, based on patients' subjective reporting of their wellbeing. Although it would be more scientifically and statistically valuable to insist on, with all former patients, and to receive updated, comprehensive, whole body imaging to confirm continued remission, expecting compliance with such a demand is not feasible. We therefore have to rely only on subjective reporting of health status by telephone. Speaking by telephone year after year with former patients who consider themselves well, whose last imaging was clear, with no further cancer treatment since leaving our clinic, have been grouped together in the category of "remission" in this study. "Assumed remission" (AR) satisfied fewer of these criteria, but involved at least stable good health of at least 6 months following cessation of our treatments. I could not reach 46 patients (Table 2, row g).

We may or may not continue gathering data for future editions of this paper, due to very little change found in the proportions and percentages of the various categories of patients year over year, as well as the increasingly labor-intensive nature of the research, as the patient population grows. However, we would like to continue try to contact all of the patients year after year, and to continue to report on each individual's outcome.

In 2015 and 2016, we changed approach, and mailed a questionnaire to each of our surviving cancer patients. Those results are described in detail in our papers "Optimal Diets for Cancer Patients."[105] and "Extroversion, Expression and Appreciation Among Cancer Patients."[106]

This paragraph summarizes Table 2, with reference herein to labelled rows of Table 2. 116 patients (rows e+g+h+i) left our practice before completing our treatments. 22 patients (row d) were killed in hospitals by medical procedures, non-cancer iatrogenic causes or simultaneous chemotherapy. The above numbers do not include any of the currently treated patients. Of the 219 patients (rows a+c+f) who were steadfast in treatment until either remission or death, 175 (row a) went into remission, and 44 patients (rows c+f) died while still our patients in our care alone. Of those 44,

12 (row f) died after a significant dietary dispute with us. The remainder is 32 patients (row c) who died while still our patients, under our care alone, following all of our protocols. This reflects a failure rate of 32 / 379 =row c / total = 8% of the total patients we treated, or a failure rate of 32 / 207 = rows c / (a+c) = 15% of the patients who were steadfast in their treatments and followed all of our recommendations. Of the 224 patients (rows a+c+i) who were steadfast in treatment, if we simply look at survivors, without confirmation of remission, then our success rate = (rows a+c+i − row c) / rows a+c+i = /[(175+32+17) − 32] / (175+32+17) =(224 − 32) / 224 = 100% - 14% = 86%.

224 steadfast patients minus 22 killed by iatrogenic causes, minus 12 who died after a dietary dispute leaves 190 patients who were steadfast and made prudent decisions. If we consider that we had 175 patients in remission of 190 who were steadfast and made prudent decisions in the treatments, then the remission rate is 92%. Late Stage IV patients tend to not do well with our treatments, although even early stage IV patients seem to have a good likelihood of going into remission.

It cannot be emphasized enough that cancer treatment has been far more effective at our clinic when patients began treatment as early as possible after diagnosis. For all stages of cancer between Stage I and early Stage IV, the success rate is between 87% and 93% (Table 5). However, for late Stage IV, the success rate has been only 29%. After a certain critical juncture of loss of vitality and overwhelming tumor burden, our treatments seem to be as unlikely to work for the patient as any other available treatment. We therefore strongly advise against a strategy of postponing natural treatments until after chemotherapy stops working.

These results must be seen in the context of when, in the course of the cancer disease process, a patient decides to, or learns of the opportunity to, embark on naturopathic treatment. The overwhelming majority of patients who come to us never heard of the possibility of such treatments until very shortly before arriving to our clinic. Therefore, we do not have the advantage of meeting the patients at the time of diagnosis, as the medical oncologists have. Rather, valuable time is often lost, and very often we only have the opportunity to begin treatment after the chemotherapy oncologist has given up on the patient. This makes our job immensely harder than it would have been if we could have started a timely treatment.

33 of 44 patients who died were Stage IV at start of treatment. This paragraph describes the ordeals of some of those individuals. One Stage IV patient had over 36 bone metastases, over 50 total metastases, and chose to have chemotherapy during our treatment (Patient #204). Four others began treatment with a tumor load that was approximately a cubic foot in the abdomen (Patients #112, 124, 301 and 356). Others chose not to follow our main dietary recommendation during the last month of their treatment, i.e. not to eat sweetened foods (Patients #264 and 275). This pancreatic cancer patient's tumors had reduced considerably during our treatments. Of the 2 pancreatic tumors, one disappeared completely, and the other shrank to approximately half the volume. This was after they had not been reduced at all by previous chemotherapy, and his oncologists had given no hope of recovery (NHR in Table 1). During this

time, the patient stayed very physically active, doing construction work in his own house at age 67. Several weeks went by, and then new pain arose. The patient then admitted to starting to eat cookies every night after dinner for the past month, which was contrary to our main dietary treatment focus, to be described below. Within 2 weeks he was dead of pancreatic cancer with new metastases. Numerous others in this group had also declined our main dietary recommendation. Another had an extensive, fast-growing inoperable glioblastoma at start of treatment, had improved briefly, then worsened and died (Patient #179). Others had cancer that our treatments simply had no effect on. Another decided to enter hospice before finishing our treatments, and we could not obtain information about how much morphine he had been given (Patient #170). And yet another had an unfortunate combination of severe constipation with fast tumor breakdown (Patient #210). This combination allows toxins to build very quickly in the body, and we could not clear them out fast enough to save her life.

Most of the late stage cancer patients who died while still only in our care arrived to our clinic very late in their disease process, years after first diagnosis, and after one of two things: 1) they had been told by an oncologist that there was no remaining hope, or 2) they had never seen an oncologist and had a growing tumor burden that had been untreated for years.

Table 3: Patients who died while only in our care prior to July 1, 2014, and stage at arrival

Stage	Total number of deceased patients, while in our care	Total patients who died despite following all of our protocols, including diet	DDD = death after dietary dispute
I	2	0	2
II	2	0	2
III	7	4	3
Early Stage IV, still functioning, activities of daily living	13	8	5
Late Stage IV, very sick, very late arrival to our clinic	20	20	0
Total	**44**	**32**	**12**

Table 4: Patients in remission or assumed remission during our care prior to July 1, 2014, and stage at arrival

Stage	Number of patients	Previous chemo-therapy with active cancer at start of our treatments	Number in each group also receiving chemo-therapy concurrently	Number in each group receiving radiation concur-rently	Number in each group receiving surgery concur-rently
I	76	5	4	6	25
II	37	1	3	2	15
III	20	6	0	1	8
Early IV	34	8	4	3	10
Late IV	8	3	1	0	1
Total	175	23	12	12	59

Table 5: Success rate by stage of cancer, for patients following all of our protocols including diet (Column 6), compared with all regardless of diet (Column 7)

1	2	3	4	5	6	7
Stage on arrival	Total patients treated until remission or death	Remission	Died, Not DDD	DDD	Remission ÷ Total = Success rate Including dietary protocol	Remission ÷ Total = Success rate** Including DDD
I	*76	76	0	2	*100%	**97%
II	*37	37	0	2	*100%	**95%
III	*24	20	4	3	*83%	**74%
Early IV	*42	34	8	5	*81%	**72%
Late IV	*28	8	20	0	*29%	**29%
Total	*207	175	32	12	*85%	**80%
Stage I through early Stage IV	*179 (not including DDD)	167	12	12	*93%	**87%

*This number does not include those who did not follow our dietary recommendations.
** These percentages in Column 7 were derived from the figures in each row of:
 [Column 3 ÷ (Column 2 + Column 5)].

Only 12 of the 175 patients we treated who went into remission also had concurrent chemotherapy (Table 4). Of all our other patients who went into remission, most had refused current chemotherapy prior to starting our treatments, although some had chosen to have it in the past. It is common for a patient who finds their way to our clinic to comment that cancer is difficult enough to endure, without the additional burden of the ill health attributable to chemotherapy alone. Our clinic's policy is never to insist that a patient either have chemotherapy or avoid it, because of the profound and severe effects on the health of such drugs, and because there is already excessive pressure on the patient by family and/or oncologists to choose one or another course of action, and because we have the utmost respect for the adult individual's inherent and self-evident right to make his/her own healthcare decisions without coercion.

Of the patients who had chemotherapy along with our treatments, all commented on feeling stronger and better able to tolerate their chemotherapy with our treatments. One patient whose tumor volume had reduced by 80% subjectively attributed this good result to both our treatments as well as chemotherapy, an evaluation that seems to defy proof or disproof (Patient #246), at least in his case.

59 of our 175 patients to go into remission also had either surgical resection or debulking of their tumors while getting our treatments. This would suggest that surgery is often a reasonable choice, perhaps even a life-saving choice, when available, and that the combination of surgical tumor resection and natural treatments was a feasible strategy for a successful outcome, although not always required for a successful outcome.

One of our patients now in remission for 6 years is and has been for years the only known survivor of Stage 3 giant cell endometrial carcinoma (Patient #306), at least according to published medical literature.[107] This remission occurred with only natural treatments after all three conventional cancer treatments, chemotherapy, radiation and surgery, were each tried multiple times and failed for this patient.

Table 6: Results for patients who left to have chemotherapy prior to 2013

Went into remission following chemotherapy	Died following chemotherapy	Not in remission, but surviving both chemotherapy and cancer as of mid-2013	Evidence of remission from our treatments alone prior to starting chemotherapy	Total who left our clinic to have chemotherapy (total of all outcomes)
4	9	5	6	24

Table 6 has not been updated since July 2013. It shows that leaving our treatments to pursue chemotherapy only possibly benefited 4 of the 24 patients who had left. However, it is possible that those 4 would have gone into remission if they had continued with our treatments alone. This table has not been updated since 2013, because a large majority of those who were thought to have left for chemotherapy could not be reached by phone. As of now, we have not attributed either pessimistic or optimistic outcomes to those we cannot reach; we simply record "NFI" in Table 1. Sometimes good or bad information comes much later. In 2014 we were absolutely delighted to welcome to our clinic visits from two cancer survivors, after only our treatments, who had not been in contact with us for 5 years and 4 years respectively (Patients #288 and 295). One lives in an RV trailer, and happened to be passing through our area again.

Table 7: Results for patients for whom the treatments had no apparent effect, as of 2013

Stage at start of treatments	Number of patients	Of these, how many had prior or current chemotherapy	Of those never having chemotx, waited years with growing mass before seeing a doctor
Stage I	1	0	0
Stage II	0	0	0
Stage III	1	0	0
Early Stage IV	4	3	1
Late Stage IV	12	6	5
Total	**18**	**9**	**6**

Table 7 shows that 15 of the 18 people for whom our treatments had no apparent effect either had prior chemotherapy or waited years with a growing mass before seeking treatment. This is likely because the patient's tumor burden became more resilient either due to the chemotherapy-imparted resistance to treatment or due to an unopposed sizeable cancer burden having the opportunity to establish an intractable stronghold in the body.

We have data for change in tumor size for relatively few patients. It must be considered that by the time a person seeks the help of a naturopathic physician for any ailment, they have often rejected, for one reason or another, the conventional medical system, leading to a distrust and disdain for conventional imaging. Imaging such as PET/CT fusion is a "hard sell" to such people. ("You want me to have radioactive glucose after telling me not to eat sugar?") Further biopsy was even less likely to be acceptable to our patients. Many of those patients left our practice for one reason or another, as discussed below, before we had any information about changing tumor size. A strong will must be present in a person to ignore the exhortations of oncologists and worried loved ones, and to pursue treatment by a naturopathic physician. This strong will easily enables rebellion against naturopathic physicians and our recommendations as well. Because we have so little information on which patients actually had increased or decreased tumor load, we have not yet had the advantage of the best way to determine the success or failure of our treatments. At present, we primarily rely on MRI imaging of the part of the torso or head or neck with the known tumor burden prior to finishing the treatments. For the blood dyscrasias, we rely on blood tests. After finishing the treatments, we recommend smaller treatments one time per month indefinitely. The local residents of course find this to be more feasible than those who temporarily moved close to our clinic for the treatments. For those who cannot pursue follow-up treatments, our contact has been one time per year with each patient, every summer, by telephone, to inquire about the current state of health from 2009 until 2014. In 2015 and 2016 we used a questionnaire instead to ask more detailed questions of our cancer survivors. However, many of the patients in remission choose to maintain an ongoing intravenous nutrient treatment one time per month. Of those patients in remission coming in for one time per month ongoing intravenous nutrient treatments, only two of those patients have come out of remission. Therefore, we recommend this strategy for all of the cancer patients who have been treated by us, as the most likely way we know of to remain in remission long-term.

There is another factor that we kept track of from July 2010 to June 2011: that year we also called people who came in to our clinic for an initial consult, but did not start our treatments. Of the 4 who visited that year, but never started our treatments, and whose family we were able to contact by phone, all four have died, according to their family members. We are no longer calling people in this category, because we are focusing our attention on the people who chose to undergo our treatments.

It cannot be assumed that those for whom our treatments failed to reduce cancer are entirely worse off. Most have described a better quality of life since starting the treatments. For example, one of the patients with stage IV breast cancer, and an increased tumor load since starting our treatments, described herself as more fit than ever since beginning our treatments, far more healthy than when she had previous chemotherapy, at 68 years old, walking 2 miles up and down hills in 22 minutes, gradually improving her time right up to the time she chose to have concurrent radiation, at which point her wellbeing, her energy, her tumor burden and her disease state began to worsen dramatically (Patient #184). Although we have not yet found the necessary combination of therapies to reduce and eliminate such a resilient cancer as hers, this patient expressed to us that the quality of life that she gained from our treatments was tangible and valuable to her.

It also cannot be assumed that conventional treatments would succeed when ours did not. For example, an ovarian cancer patient (Patient #112) was persuaded by family members to stop our treatments and resume chemotherapy, even though chemotherapy had not eliminated her cancer in the past, and our subsequent treatments did in fact reduce the tumors to a fraction of their original size, in only a fraction of the usual treatment time. When this patient complied with her family members and resumed chemotherapy, the remaining tumor mass grew again, steadily through two months of chemotherapy. The oncologist then gave up and offered her no more chemotherapy and directed her to hospice care. A number of other patients also did very well in measures of tumor size and wellbeing with our treatments. Then in some cases, chemotherapy oncologists or family members persuaded or pressured or coerced the patient to have chemotherapy instead. Usually, that patient then quickly declined and died.

For the 116 patients who decided to leave before finishing our treatments, it is difficult to assess the degree of success or failure. Reasons for leaving were often not given. There was sometimes a phone message requesting to cancel the future appointments without explanation. However, when we were told reasons for leaving, the following were common:

1) Financial reasons: no insurance reimbursement made it hard to continue paying for our treatments out of pocket. This was by far the most common reason given. This was expected to change in 2014 when the Affordable Care Act mandated insurance reimbursement of naturopathic medicine, to the best of our understanding, under new private insurance plans. However, that mandate has not yet been implemented. Some insurance companies were much better about reimbursing for naturopathic medicine than others.

2) The patient did not feel that anything important was happening with the treatment. There was a strange viewpoint expressed by some patients that cancer is not very frightening, once they saw that they, as well as all of the other non-chemotherapy cancer patients in our IV rooms maintained their vitality, their hair and their bodily functions, and almost always with improved fitness. This led some to the dangerously wrong conclusion that cancer was easy to conquer, could probably have happened at home with store-bought nutrients, and that our treatments had not accomplished much, and perhaps had not even contributed to their continued wellbeing, and that they would have remained well anyway.

3) A related viewpoint was that improvement in the patient's condition should have been faster and more dramatic. If the condition seemingly stayed the same, some patients viewed this as evidence of failure, of not defeating cancer fast enough, and concluded that the treatment was not working, and that they should not waste any

more time or money pursuing it, and that it was time to leave and explore other avenues.

4) Family members or oncologists disapproved of natural cancer treatment and persuasively urged chemotherapy exclusively.

5) The patient had traveled from another state to receive our treatments, but wanted to return home to be with family, regardless of expected outcome.

*Table 8: Summary of quality of life changes, as of July 2011, by assessment of naturopathic physician along with patient self-evaluation during naturopathic care of the patients whose wellbeing stayed the same or improved prior to July 2011

Quality of life changes	Number of patients	Number in each group who went into remission	Number in each group also receiving chemotherapy
Came in with high wellbeing / Still the same way	92	70	3
Came in occupationally functional but not physically fit /Ultimately improved vitality	34	25	3
Came in occupationally functional but not physically fit / Still the same way	17	3	4
Total	143	98	10

*Note: This table has not been updated since the 2011 edition of this paper, due to the labor-intensive nature of this research, and not much expected change in proportion of the different groups.

If one considers quality of life as a criterion for success, then of the patients who stayed well or got better during our treatments, 143 patients out of 165 who had come to us prior to July 2011, make a success rate of 87%. For most of the remaining 13% of total patients, they mostly came to us after exhausting all conventional cancer treatments and were mostly late stage 4, or had other co-morbidities. These co-morbidities included: pulmonary fibrosis, asbestosis, uranium poisoning, radiation poisoning, more than 15 CT scans done on one individual, chronic antibiotic-resistant infections, Clostridium difficile, scleroderma, cirrhosis, pneumonia, asthma, diabetes, rapid tumor breakdown with poor elimination, radiation illness, chemotherapy intolerance, complications from previous surgery, blood clots where the tumor had compressed multiple veins before the tumor was eliminated, hepatic coma.

Table 9: Patients choosing to have monthly follow-up treatments

	Stage	Cancer	C	R	S	CANCER OUTCOME	WELL-BEING
1	2	breast	No	No	Yes	R	HFwE/Job
2	2	lung	No	No	No	R x years. Now battling Valley Fever.	HfwE/Job
3	3	breast	No	No	Yes	R	Hf/Sa
4	4	breast	No	No PR	No PS	R	HF/Sa
5	1	breast	No	No	Yes	R	HFwE/Job
6	1	breast	No	No	Yes	R	HfwE (15 mi bike rides)/ Sa
7	2	breast	No	No	No	R. Current	Imp; HfwE
8	1	Walden-strom's lymphoma	No	No	No	Numbers go up and down with allergens, but much better strength now	Imp mostly; strenuous exercise, recrea-tional travel
9	4	uterine	No	No	Yes	R	
10	2 NHR	breast	No	No	Yes	R	HFwE/ Sa
11	1	breast	No	No	Yes	R	HFwE/Sa/ Job
12	4	ovarian and peritoneal	No	No	Yes	R x 3 years, then recurrence	HFwE/Imp
13	2	breast	No	No	Yes	R	HfwE/Job
14	1	prostate	No	No	No	R	HFwE/Sa/ Job
15	4 NHR	ovarian	No	No	Yes	Rx 3 years	HFwE in 80's
16	2	breast	No	No	Yes	R	HfwE
17	4	colon	No	No	No PS	R	HF/Sa/ retired
18	4	breast	No	No	Yes	R	HF
19	1	breast	Yes	Yes	Yes	R	HfwE, Job
20	4	ALL leukemia	No PC	No	No	R x 4 years	Imp, HFwE
21	1	breast	No	No	Yes	R	HF
22	3	breast	No	No	Yes	R	HF/Job
23	2	breast	No	No	Yes PS	R, then recurrence, then lumpectomy. Current.	HFwE, Sa
24	2	breast	No	No	Yes		R| HFwE/ Imp

25	3 NHR	giant cell endometrial	No, PC	No, PR	Debulking but not resection PS	R x 5 years	Imp/HF wE/Job
26	1	breast	No	No	Yes	R	HFw/E, strenuous; "boot camp"
27	1	bladder	No	No	No	R	HfwE/Job
28	3	breast	No	No	Yes	R	HF

Summary of table of follow-up treatments: Total pts. = 28. Total still in remission = 26 = 93% of total.

It is important to note that not all of the patients did all that was recommended by us. For example, although we recommend beginning our treatments immediately after diagnosis, almost all patients delayed naturopathic treatment for months to years after initial diagnosis of cancer, mostly due to lack of information to the public about the effectiveness of natural treatments for cancer. The enormous disadvantage of such delay to the naturopathic physician's work and effectiveness cannot be overstated. Chemotherapy is known to impart a resilience to tumors that makes it hard for any subsequent treatment to have an effect. It is surprising that our success has been as high as it is, given the severe disadvantage of beginning natural treatments months to years after cancer has had a head start in its growth and takeover of the body, as well as the debilitation of the general health of the patient.

Other patients chose to disregard the dietary recommendations that we made or to only observe the recommendations partially. Others chose to have fewer in-office treatments than were recommended. Others decided to choose only some of the recommended treatments due to financial constraints

110

or inconvenience. However, as our clinic has demonstrated longer, sustained success with an ever-increasing number of patients, and a majority obviously well patients are present and visible in our clinic on our busiest workdays, and the value of our treatment protocols become obvious to more and more visitors to our clinic, both patients and their family members, compliance with our recommendations has generally been much better during the last few years than previously, with regard to both diet and on-site treatments.

Some of the patients who came out of remission had discontinued our main dietary recommendation. This was especially disappointing to us because for example, Patient #307, after being out of contact for almost two years after going into remission, called to inform us that she was now physically active and had at last stopped smoking. (She had smoked all through our treatments.) She had gone off of the diet, and then developed recurrence of cancer and died.   Another patient (Patient #49) went quickly back into remission.

Most patients chose not to follow our recommendation to have monthly follow-up treatments after remission. But of those who did, 28 patients, 26 of them are still in remission. That is 93%.

Discussion

175 patients went into remission by mid-2014 during our treatments of a total of 207 up to that time who complied with all of our treatment protocols until either remission or death. This is 175 / 207 = 85% success over all stages and all types of cancer. For Stages I

through early Stage IV, it is 167 / 179 (remission / total) = 93% success rate. If we consider that only 175 patients went into remission, out of the total 379 patients who had our treatment for at least two weeks prior to mid-2014, then only 175 / 379 = 46% have gone into remission, which is quite low. However, the 379 number includes those who only had sporadic treatments, and those who ignored our dietary and exercise recommendations, and those who were killed by chemotherapy and other iatrogenic procedures. Therefore, we do not consider the 46% as representative of what happens with patients who follow our recommendations steadfastly, and therefore does not reflect the work of our clinic. If one considers those who were steadfast in their treatments and died, divided by all who were steadfast in their treatments, then the failure rate is 32 / 207 = 15% of the patients who were steadfast in their treatments and followed all of our recommendations. Of the 224 patients who were steadfast in treatment, if we simply look at survivors, without confirmation of remission, then our success rate = (224 – 32) / 224 = 86%.

Numerous natural agents were simultaneously employed to reduce or inactivate or necrose or eliminate human neoplasms in vivo. We chose to use these agents together because cancer is a multifactorial disease and has not yet been fought effectively in a majority of patients with a single agent. Specific combinations of natural substances were chosen with regard to the type of cancer and circumstances of each individual cancer patient. Licensed naturopathic physicians are well-qualified to design such treatment programs because of our broad and extensive training with natural and conventional substances and how to combine them. Because of our unprecedented and consistent success in treating cancer since 2006, we believe we have demonstrated the need for simultaneous well-tolerated cancer-disrupting treatments.

Successful outcomes were more likely with steadfast patient compliance during the entire duration of the treatment process. Although our results are a strong improvement over any other cancer treatment protocols that we have found, both conventional and natural, if measured by either patient remission or survival, these treatment strategies are still not adequate to eliminate all patients' cancers and must be further developed.

Chapter 8

Glycemic restriction in cancer patients:
A 7-year, controlled interventional study

Abstract

Background
Previous research has shown a correlation between blood sugar or glycemic load and cancer growth for a number of types of cancer. Those studies were retrospective and/or studies of fewer than 20 human subjects and/or studies on mice. This study is a 7-year interventional study of 317 human patients at one clinic, who were treated naturopathically, with anti-neoplastic nutrients and herbs, plus the recommended dietary intervention of abstention from sweetened foods.

Methods
We analyzed the clinical significance (mortality) of sweetened food consumption among cancer patients at our clinic. Since 2006, this clinic has collected data on sugar consumption in cancer patients, and has actively recommended, but never enforced in any way,

avoiding the consumption of sweetened foods (except with the sweetener Stevia rebaudiana, which has no sugar content or sugar alcohol content). In this controlled interventional study, we followed the diets and outcomes of all 317 cancer patients who came to our clinic with a diagnosis of cancer, and who stayed at least two weeks in our care. All results are reported in this paper.

Results
The remission rate is significantly different for the following two categories: all patients: 151 / 317 = 48% and those who ate sweetened foods: 9 / 29 = 31%. However, the difference in these two groups is much more pronounced if we consider those patients who continued our treatments until either remission or death. Comparing all patients who were steadfast in our recommended naturopathic treatments with the sweetened food eaters who were steadfast in all but dietary recommendations, 151 / 183 = 83% of all totally steadfast patients went into remission, but only 9 / 25 = 36% of the steadfast sweetened food eaters went into remission.

Of all patients who were steadfast in the treatments (including our sweetened food eaters), 32 / 183 = 17% died while still under our care, but considering only the sweetened food eaters who were otherwise steadfast in the treatments, 16 / 25 = 64% died.

Conclusion
Consuming sweetened foods (other than stevia sweetened foods) made a significant difference in patient outcome across all stages and all types of cancer. We therefore recommend that the diet of cancer patients not contain sweetened foods other than stevia.

Background and Methods

We analyzed the clinical significance (mortality) of sweetened food consumption among cancer patients. Since 2006, this clinic has collected data on sugar consumption in cancer patients, and has actively recommended, but never enforced in any way, abstention from the consumption of sweetened foods. This clinic has no inpatient facilities and no food service. All patients chose all of their own food, all of which originated from outside this clinic. Data from all 317 patients who came to us with a diagnosis of cancer are included in this interventional study, excluding only those cancer patients who decided against further treatment after less than two weeks in our care.

We treated with natural methods alone, choosing among methods with research-established anti-neoplastic effect, both oral and intravenous, dietary and supplemented, nutritional and herbal, having a preference for those with high patient tolerance and compatibility, and varying with individual needs and tolerance, according to the standard naturopathic principle of "Treat the whole person."

Dietary interventions are of the utmost importance in cancer therapy, especially keeping blood sugar low. Most of the research on the subject establishes a correlation between blood glucose and tumor growth. Using PET imaging preferentially for tumor evaluation, clinicians make use of the fact that tumors take up blood glucose disproportionately over benign tissue, which implies an especially glucose-dependent metabolism in cancer cells. In fact, the difference between uptake of glucose in a malignant tumor and uptake in normal tissue is so stark that the rough outlines of a tumor may be seen on a PET simply from the borders of where glucose uptake is strong next to where it is weak.

Research has shown a correlation between blood sugar or glycemic load and cancer growth for pancreatic cancer,[108] [109] [110] [111] breast cancer,[112] [113] [114] [115] prostate cancer,[116] [117] gastric cancer, [118] [119] colorectal cancer,[120] [121] [122] [123] ovarian cancer,[124] [125] endometrial cancer,[126] [127] and liver and biliary tract cancers.[128] [129] Given all of this evidence, it would be reckless for a physician to allow a cancer patient to assume that sugar intake is harmless. We therefore ask all of our cancer patients to avoid sweeteners, such as sugar, honey, maple syrup, corn syrup, high fructose corn syrup, alcohol, alcohol sugars and plant nectars, as well as fruit juices, because such foods tend to have the highest glycemic indices. Use of stevia is encouraged if and when a sweetener is desired. For the same reason, we asked patients to also limit other refined carbohydrates, specifically flour products.

Whole natural foods: vegetables, fruits, whole grains, eggs, dairy and other animal proteins are encouraged as the entire diet, with the widest available variety in those groups. Many patients arrive to our clinic already consuming all of those types of foods. Others arrive with different diets. Some patients have chosen a vegan diet. Others have chosen an ovo-lacto-vegetarian diet. Many others are omnivores. Others avoid grains altogether. We have not actively pushed our patients to one or the other of these diets, because we tried to maintain the primary dietary focus on the avoidance of sweeteners, without distraction by other dietary priorities. Keeping the focus exclusively on the avoidance of sweeteners seems to minimize the opportunity to forget that one guideline. Patients may eat absolutely anything they like, except that we strongly urge the avoidance of sweeteners, except for Stevia rebaudiana, which has no significant sugar content. Through repeated reminding, with gentle, encouraging consultation and troubleshooting of sugar cravings, as well as brainstorming of alternative foods that may satisfy those cravings, during patient consults, we create a situation where our patients are unlikely to completely forget our recommendation when given a choice of whether to have dessert or skip dessert.

The overwhelming influence of the oncology profession on diet has suppressed this type of recommendation among many physicians. Chemotherapy IV rooms are known for having candy dishes in plain sight. Most oncologists have generally recommended that cancer patients eat desserts so intently that it seems the patients' primary responsibility is to keep their weight up, without regard for specific health effects of various foods. Under this sugar-oriented food culture, both in the American culture at large and in the oncology clinic, other physicians less specifically credentialed to treat cancer patients shrink from challenging this dictum of the oncologists.

However, back when we started this dietary recommendation to our cancer patients in 2006, the time was already more than ripe to rebel against the sweet-tooth trend, because most of the above-cited research on sugar consumption and tumor growth had already been published. So at our clinic we decided to acknowledge the little known but already well-established connection between sugar and cancer, and thus to recommend sugar avoidance to our cancer patients.

Sugar and its effect on the body

So let's look at what we mean by "sugar." Commonly the word "sugar" means sucrose, derived from sugar cane. Sucrose, a disaccharide, is a compound of glucose and fructose, each a monosaccharide, and sugar is composed equally of both. High-fructose corn syrup is similar, except that it has a higher proportion of fructose to glucose. 80% of sucrose used worldwide is from cane sugar; most of the rest is from beets. It is already common knowledge that sugar is "empty calories," that is, no protein or fat or complex carbohydrates. In its refined form it contains no nutrients at all, no vitamins, minerals, flavonoids or other antioxidants, no fiber, no amino acids. However, sugar is far more damaging to the health than simply the null effect of empty calories.

Epidemiologically, sugar consumption was thought be 40 pounds per person per year in the U.S. in 1986.[130] By the early 2000s, Americans were consuming 90 pounds per person per year, which coincided with the time that one-third of Americans were obese and 14 million were diabetic.[131] The most likely explanation of this correlation is that sudden intake of a large amount of sugar overwhelms the liver, which then turns excess sugar to fat, primarily palmitate – a saturated fatty acid, and puts triglycerides in the bloodstream. This process is also thought to correlate with insulin resistance, as I'll discuss below.

Population studies have corroborated these findings in various countries, but the idea that sugar could be deleterious to the health fell into disfavor in the 1970s, as American nutritionists at that time followed en masse Ancel Keys and his Seven Countries Study. This study, implicating saturated fat in cardiovascular disease, had actually been a 22-country study, in which those countries that contradicted the hypothesis were quietly dropped from the discussion.

Incidentally, those same countries were found to have a direct relationship between sugar consumption and heart disease, but that was not the widely-publicized conclusion. Saturated fat became the scapegoat. In the following decades, salt would come to play the role of villain. As country after country fell victim to the damaging effects of sugar in the diet, one scapegoat after another took the blame. The British physiologist John Yudkin found an effect of sugar consumption on obesity, diabetes and cardiovascular disease,[132] and brought the public's attention to the health effects of sucrose in his 1972 book Pure, White and Deadly.[133] Yudkin was often personally attacked, quite virulently, for writing about the pathological conditions either caused by or worsened by sugar. In 1975, William Dufty challenged the conventional thinking on sugar with his bestseller Sugar Blues.[134] Then Nancy Appleton wrote "141 Reasons Sugar Ruins Your Health,"[135] and Lick the Sugar Habit.[136] In the last few years, Robert Lustig has explained the widespread damage in a way that the public is beginning to appreciate. But the best at breaking down the chemistry to clear language as well as the politics, intrigue and history of American food fights is journalist Gary Taubes, author of "Is Sugar Toxic?"[137] as well as the decade-old but still current "What If It's All Been A Big, Fat Lie?"[138] and "Why We Get Fat."[139]

Sugar is broken down in the duodenum by sucrase and isomaltase glycoside hydrolases. A rapid rise in blood glucose quickly follows ingestion of pure sucrose, or sucrose-rich solids and especially liquids. Sweets accompanied by fats, proteins or fiber will enter the bloodstream slower than sweets alone in a refined carbohydrate vehicle, such as a cookie. But whether fast or slow, insulin is secreted by the pancreas in response to the presence of sugar in the blood. A lot of sudden sugar in the blood results in a lot of insulin secreted by the pancreas. When that happens too much or for too many years, the pancreas becomes depleted and can't keep up with the body's demand for insulin. Blood sugar rises beyond normal range, leading to a Type II diabetes diagnosis. In animal studies of sugar bingeing this process began in only a few weeks.[140] Chronically high insulin has other effects besides diabetes: atherosclerosis and hypertension, and unfavorable HDL / LDL ratios.

In order to understand the relationship of this to cancer, first, we have to look at epidemiology again. The WHO International Agency for Research on Cancer found that cancer is more prevalent in populations where there is obesity, diabetes and metabolic syndrome.[141] The likely cause and effect is that sugar consumption causes insulin secretion, and that insulin, as well as its closely related hormone, insulin-like growth factor, promotes tumor growth. One effect of IGF-1 is to deliver sugar into a cell, among other things. However, very high protein diets can also result in elevated IGF-1. It can bind to insulin receptors, and like insulin, the receptor for IGF-1 is a receptor tyrosine kinase. Too much IGF-1 can result in a transient hypoglycemia. IGF-1 acts as a growth factor in breast cancer,[142] prostate cancer,[143] and lung cancer,[144] among other cancers.

Tumor growth is thought to occur by the fact that insulin delivers sugar to cells and that cancer cells are thought to be more dependent on sugar than normal cells. Whereas normal cells down-regulate their receptors after a certain level of saturation with sugar, cancer appears to be insatiable. Cancer's rapid growth seems to place no limit on the sugar it can use. Insulin delivers that sugar. Some cells develop mutations to enhance insulin's influence on the cell's sugar uptake. Craig Thompson MD, President of Memorial Sloan Kettering Cancer Center in New York has studied insulin and IGF's influence on cancer cells and has said he believes that insulin is what drives malignant tumors to take up more and more blood sugar and to metabolize it, and that it is this process that allows many pre-cancerous cells to undergo the mutations that make them malignant.[145]

But what do cancer cells get from sugar that is so useful to their growth? We know that sugar provides quick energy, and that not a lot of processing needs to happen before the body and brain use sugar as fuel. Cancer grows faster than normal tissue, so we can see the expedience of using sugar as a fuel. But unlike normal cells, cancer can live where there is little oxygen. So instead of a normal metabolism, that is cellular respiration, cancer cells preferentially undergo anaerobic fermentation, which converts NADH to NAD+, which then enables anaerobic or aerobic glycolysis. Otto Warburg discovered this difference between normal and malignant cells in 1924.[146] Initially, he thought that all cancer cells used only anaerobic glycolysis to produce energy, but it is now known that cancer is capable of both kinds of metabolism. The beginning and end is that cancer cells convert sugar to lactic acid. No oxygen means no electron transport chain. Even in the presence of adequate oxygen levels, cancer cells seem to default to fermentation rather than oxidative phosphorylation to produce ATP, although ATP is formed much more efficiently from the electron transport chain and oxidative phosphorylation than with fermentation. For the large amount of sugar metabolized in fermentation, little ATP is formed. It may be the case that because this fermentation process is so inefficient in its production of ATP that only large amounts of sugar and a high rate of sugar uptake will work to drive rapid tumor growth, and this is likely why cancer is so dependent on the presence of sugar.

Does this mean that starving the cancer cell of sugar kills the cancer cell? Cancer patients on a ketogenic diet, which is an extremely low carbohydrate diet, have been observed to fare well. To summarize the classic ketogenic diet, fat outweighs the total of protein and carbohydrates 4 to 1 by weight, and total carbohydrates is limited to 20 to 40 grams per day. The classic ketogenic diet eliminates simple and complex carbohydrates: sweeteners, fruits, grains, and starchy vegetables. A later development adds medium-chain triglycerides, such as coconut oil, and a little more variety in the proteins and carbohydrates than the classic ketogenic diet. The lack of carbohydrates in this diet makes metabolism default to burning fats for energy. The liver converts fat to fatty acids and ketone bodies, which the brain can use as fuel in the absence of glucose. A study of ketogenic diet in animal models of glioma found various effects that made glioma cells behave more like normal cells.[147]   On the gross level in animal studies, a ketogenic diet was found either to reduce the tumor size or slow tumor growth in glioblastoma,[148] prostate cancer,[149] gastric cancer,[150] and lung cancer.[151]   It was also found to improve quality of life in patients with advanced metastatic disease in a variety of cancers.[152]

From these observations, we may not be able to jump all the way to the conclusion that sugar causes cancer, or even that the elimination of sugar eliminates cancer. However, we can certainly become alert to a cancer patient's risks in continuing the consumption of sugar, and the possible benefit from eliminating it from the diet.

Results

Regarding the patients at our clinic, 29 patients acknowledged to us that they had disregarded or somehow not adhered to our main dietary recommendation; that is, that they ate sweetened foods at some time during their treatment. The doctors and staff try never to have a judgmental approach to our patients. If a patient has acknowledged that he or she has not abstained from sweets entirely, then we take a co-responsible (some might call it co-dependent) approach. We take responsibility for not having sufficiently encouraged or offered ideas for adequate and satisfactory substitutes for sweetened foods. So then during one-on-one consults we try to offer more, and more individually applicable, suggestions for the sweet cravings. For example, one person may be more drawn to alcohol, while another is more drawn to chocolate. Yet another may have a coffee habit in which coffee tastes bad to them without sugar. For others, it is ice cream that they want. Whether we were successful or not in persuading such individuals to adopt our recommended diet, we report that category of patient below as one who disregarded our dietary recommendation, unless they agreed to give up sweets at the beginning of treatment and stayed steadfast in that diet.

Our data is reported as of July 1, 2013. 20 patients died while still exclusively in our care, following all of our protocols, including dietary. These were all types of cancer and all stages of cancer, especially the more advanced stages. 12 more died while still in our care, but having ignored one of our main treatment recommendations, that is to avoid sweetened foods. 16 of our cancer patients have come out of remission. 5 of those are now back in remission. 4 of those 16 had discontinued our main dietary recommendation.

Table 1: Summarized outcomes of naturopathic management of 317 cancer cases

Outcome	Number of patients	Number in each group also receiving chemotherapy	Number in each group also receiving surgery
Remission or assumed remission	151	7	47
Died while still only in our care, following all of our protocols and diet	20	0	1
Iatrogenic death in hospitals or by MDs	20	14	7
Of those who left before finishing treatment, number who died after leaving (except for DDD)*	46	1	10
Death after dietary dispute	12	1	2
Still being treated, not yet in remission	18	3	10
No current information but never known to be in remission	33	3	9
Waiting to know status, or conflicting information	17	0	2
Total	317	29	88

* DDD: death after dietary dispute.

Table 2: Summarized outcomes of naturopathic management of 29 cancer cases in which there was a dietary dispute regarding sweetened food consumption

Outcome	Number of patients	Number in each group also receiving chemo-therapy	Number in each group also receiving surgery
Remission or assumed remission	9	0	5
Died while still only in our care, following all of our protocols	0	0	0
Iatrogenic death in hospitals or by MDs	1	0	0
Of those who left before finishing treatment, number who died after leaving (except for DDD)*	0	0	0
Death after dietary dispute	12	1	2
Still being treated, not yet in remission	0	0	0
No current information but never known to be in remission	7	2	0
Waiting to know status, or conflicting information	0	0	0
Total	**29**	**3**	**7**

* DDD: death after dietary dispute.

Table 3: Summarized outcomes of naturopathic management of 288 cancer cases, all of whom were able to avoid consumption of sweeteners

Outcome	Number of patients	Number in each group also receiving chemo-therapy	Number in each group also receiving surgery
Remission or assumed remission	142	7	42
Died while still only in our care, following all of our protocols and diet	20	0	1
Iatrogenic death in hospitals or by MDs	19	14	7
Of those who left before finishing treatment, number who died after leaving (except for DDD)*	46	1	10
Death after dietary dispute	0	0	0
Still being treated, not yet in remission	18	3	10
No current information but never known to be in remission	26	1	9
Waiting to know status, or conflicting information	17	0	2
Total	**288**	**26**	**81**

* DDD: death after dietary dispute.

Tables 1, 2 and 3 show comparable information for three groups of patients: Table 1 summarizes all patients who presented to our clinic for cancer treatment, and who stayed in our treatments for at least two weeks. Table 2 shows the same information for those who chose to eat sweetened foods. Table 3 shows the same information for those who chose to avoid sweetened foods. The remission rate is different for all patients: 151 / 317 = 48% and those who ate sweetened foods: 9 / 29 = 31% and those who avoided sweetened foods: 142 / 288 = 49%. However, the difference in these three groups is even more pronounced if we consider those patients who stayed with our treatments until either remission or death, as in Tables 4, 5 and 6.

Table 4: Steadfast patients, by stage of cancer – all patients

Stage	Total patients treated until remission or death	Remission	Died	Remission / Total = Success rate
I	65	64	1	98%
II	30	29	1	97%
III	17	14	3	82%
Early IV	49	37	12	76%
Late IV	22	7	15	32%
Total	**183**	**151**	**32***	**83%**
Stage I through early Stage IV	**161**	**144**	**17 (including DDD)**	**89%**

*This number includes those who did not follow our dietary recommendations.

Table 5: Steadfast patients, by stage of cancer – sweet eaters

Stage	Total patients treated until remission or death	Remission	Died	Remission / Total = Success rate
I	5	4	1	80%
II	4	3	1	75%
III	3	0	3	0%
Early IV	10	2	8	20%
Late IV	3	0	3	0%
Total	25	9	16	36%
Stage I through early Stage IV	22	9	13	41%

Table 6: Steadfast patients, by stage of cancer – sweetener avoiders

Stage	Total patients treated until remission or death	Remission	Died	Remission / Total = Success rate
I	60	60	0	**100%**
II	26	26	0	**100%**
III	14	14	0	**100%**
Early IV	39	35	4	**90%**
Late IV	19	7	12	**37%**
Total	**158**	**142**	**16**	**90%**
Stage I through early Stage IV	**139**	**135**	**4**	**97%**

Comparing all patients who were steadfast in the treatments (Table 4) with the sweetened food eaters, who were steadfast in all but dietary recommendations (Table 5), we see that 151 / 183 = 83% went into remission, but only 9 / 25 = 36% of the sweetened food eaters went into remission. 90% of the steadfast patients who avoided sweeteners went into remission.

Of all patients who were steadfast in the treatments, (including our sweetened food eaters), 32 / 183 = 17% died, but considering only the sweetened food eaters who were otherwise steadfast in the treatments, 16 / 25 = 64% died. Of the steadfast patients who avoided sweeteners, 16 / 158 = 10% died.

Conclusion

Consuming sweetened foods (other than stevia sweetened foods) made a significant difference in patient outcome across both all stages and all types of cancer among patients presenting to our clinic. We therefore recommend that the diet of cancer patients not contain sweeteners other than stevia.

Chapter 9

Metabolic theory of cancer and common misconceptions

Oncology as a field is very resistant to change, so much so that the vast majority of research scientists and oncologists working in this area still believe in a notion that has been soundly disproven several times during the last century.

I am talking about the Somatic Mutation Theory of Cancer (SMT), which reached its heyday in 1976. This was a time that various research efforts had arrived at common conclusions and then convinced the world of a dogma that has taken stubborn hold ever since. That dogma says this:

Cancer is caused by damage to DNA, which leads to damaged genes. Those genes, oncogenes, are responsible for the reproduction of cancer cell lines (which one could think of as multi-generation families), which grow unchecked to the point of being a tumor. Those tumors can be tested for damaged genes and will allegedly show those genes.

Not only has this particular dogma been proven to be false, or at most only true a tiny percentage of the time in a tiny percentage of the cells of a tumor, but this particular dogma has launched the confetti of pink ribbons all over the Western world and billions of dollars chasing those ribbons in pursuit of research for a now-failed theory.

Why is the SMT wrong? Don't you get cancer when your DNA is damaged or when you inherited bad genes? Here is the problem: The genetic machinery is in the nucleus of a cell. Studies have shown that if you transplant a cancer nucleus into a normal cell, the cell stays normal. But if you transplant the mitochondria, the power plant so to speak, of a cancer cell into a normal cell, then you get a cancer cell as a result.

In other words, the mitochondria (energy supplier) is decisive. The nucleus (genetic library) is not decisive in creating or maintaining a cancer cell.

Therefore, it is NOT the genetic machinery, not the nucleus, which creates cancer. It is damage to the mitochondria that creates the cancer. Two groups working independently of each other found this to be the case. One was at the University of Vermont, and the other at the University of Texas, Southwestern Medical Center in Dallas. Both research teams confirmed in repeated experiments that putting a cancer nucleus into normal cells results in normal cells, but putting cancerous cytoplasm (which contain the cells' mitochondria) into normal cells results in cancerous cells nearly every time. These results were independently verified to be the same nearly every time.[153] [154] [155] [156]

The implications of this research are enormous: It means that the determining factor in creating cancer is not in the nucleus where the genetic material is. Rather, the decisive factor in creating cancer is in the cytoplasm where the mitochondria are. Cancer arises from this and this alone: impaired cellular respiration. Cellular respiration is known to occur in the mitochondria.

The genetic damage that happens to a cell is simply one of the results of the original cause, which is damaged mitochondria. Later I will discuss damaged mitochondria.

Many billions of dollars of research money went into the Cancer Genome Atlas (TGCA) Project funded by the National Cancer Institute (NCI), which purported to identify the cancerous genes in tumors. It is a multi-national project so ambitious in scope that writer Travis Christofferson calls it the Manhattan Project of cancer.[157] But something went terribly wrong. The genetic makeup of one part of a tumor is different almost every time from the genetic make-up of another part of even the same tumor! [158]

In other words, any pursuit of a genetic signature or genetic identification of a tumor is a waste of time, because it only relates to a small part of that tumor. There is no single, coherent genetic characterization of a person's cancer, and almost every type of genetic variation can be found within the cancerous tissue of one person. That is, there is no reliable or consistent genetic signature to a person's cancer. [159] [160] [161] In other words, all that money collected for cancer research has been donated, and is still being donated, to a now disproven theory.

There are scientists involved in the TCGA project who now realize its failure, and are acknowledging the "sobering realization" that "maybe it is just too hard to figure out." Of the roughly 700 drugs to come out of the TCGA, none were helpful to patients, except perhaps Gleevec, which actually seems to be something of a metabolic drug, rather than a SMT-type drug. The drugs that came out of these research efforts generally offer the patient no greater duration of life and certainly no greater quality of life.

This particular realization, though it has now become apparent to some cancer researchers, is not the headline-making news that it ought to be, because the embarrassment and financial loss of the funding of the gene theory / SMT would be devastating to pink ribboners and the like. The disgrace also of having to admit that decades of work were a complete mistake, and that all the money donated in that direction had been an utter waste, would be a bit hard for anyone to take, not to mention would stir up the pitchfork temperaments of the public who has donated so generously over the years, and may very well feel that a refund is in order. So, sparing all that anguish, the status quo does not get disrupted. The bigger loss of course is the lives of cancer patients who were sold the bill of goods that later betrayed them and cost them their lives.

As a result of finding different genetic signatures in different parts of the same tumor, researchers who subscribe relentlessly to the SMT have then concluded this: That cancer is such a complex array of diseases that we are further from understanding cancer than at any time in the past. The assumption then is that cancer is not one disease but many different diseases in a complex array, but that it must – because they have always been told it must – be related to and caused by genetic aberrations. This results in a further assumption, that the complexity of cancer makes it almost unknowable. This is a faulty premise, and an unnecessary one, if the majority of cancer researchers had not been so eager to dismiss Nobel prize-winning biochemist Otto Warburg's findings, which have been verified throughout the world and over the 90 years since he announced them, and which I will discuss below.

The fact is, and I am by no means the first to say it, is that the genetic paradigm is deeply flawed. Groupthink sclerosed over a long-cherished dogma, and hardened so relentlessly that it is still considered blasphemy to question the idea of the genetic origins of cancer. Yet this insistence on the familiar dogma prevents new information – as well as new confirmation of very old information – from coming to the fore and getting a fair hearing.

Let's start at the beginning: The scientist who first understood cancer well was Otto Warburg, the world's leading biochemist and a Nobel laureate. In 1924 he figured out the essential nature of cancer:

> "Cancer, above all other diseases, has countless secondary causes. But, even for cancer, there is only one prime cause. Summarized in a few words, the prime cause of cancer is the replacement of the

respiration of oxygen in normal body cells by a fermentation of sugar."[162]

Because of the many secondary causes, and also because cancer could take root in any tissue of the body, Warburg concluded what should be obvious to all, that cancer is not a peripheral problem.

Rather cancer is a very fundamental problem. Therefore, it is a problem of the basic mechanism of the body: metabolism. What is metabolism? It is an economy so to speak in which the currency is units of energy, molecules and macromolecules or nutrients. Warburg hit on the true nature of cancer: a disorder that is at the very essence of how we function. Forget genetic changes; those come afterward, and are not decisive, not helpful to the basic understanding of cancer nor to its cure.

Otto Warburg's thesis did not find much favor in his time, and even less after his death in 1970. If it weren't for research scientists Pete Pedersen and Young Hee Ko of Johns Hopkins University School of Medicine taking an interest in and testing Warburg's theory [163] through the 1970's and 1980's, Warburg's findings may well have been completely forgotten. Yet through the work of Pedersen, Ko and then Thomas Seyfried, whose book Cancer as a Metabolic Disease[164], establishes and gathers the empirical studies that proved Warburg correct, we now have a substantial body of proof in favor of Warburg's theory.

Another very helpful work, especially to laypeople wanting to sort through the science is Travis Christofferson's Tripping Over The Truth.[165]

Seyfried in particular was able to show evidence confirming Warburg's metabolic theory, that damage to the mitochondria, the engines of the cell, rather than the nucleus where the genetic material lies, was the decisive factor in whether a cell turned cancerous or not. He was able to show that the genetic damage that we see in cancer cells is not the cause of the cancer, but rather one of the secondary effects of this damage to the mitochondria.

When mitochondria are damaged, they send distress signals to the nucleus of the cell, and it is only then that we see the hallmark features of cancer: genetic instability, uncontrolled growth, cell immortality, etc. But these are only downstream effects, the very effects that the multi-billion dollar cancer research industry assumed were causative, which wasted an enormous amount of resources, and delayed what could have been life-saving understanding of cancer for generations of cancer patients.

Back in the 1920's, Otto Warburg reasoned that cancer must be fundamentally different from most other diseases. Whereas other diseases damage a predictable part of the body or body system, cancer on the other hand, could arise just about anywhere. Therefore, he reasoned it must be a more fundamental disease, not having to do with a function of a part of the body, as the other diseases. But rather it had to do with something much more basic, as we said before: that is, metabolism.

First, let's talk about cells. Cells are a basic operational unit in living things. They take in nutrients, and perform work, with division of labor, in various cell parts, called organelles, and produce and discharge waste. They take signals and information and direction from inside and outside the cell. Mitochondria are of particular interest here, because the hundreds of mitochondria in each cell are the furnaces or energy plants of the cell. Oxygen is essential to mitochondrial health and function. Lack of oxygen disrupts them, and prolonged lack of oxygen causes permanent damage and death to mitochondria. Okay, let's store that away, because Otto Warburg did not yet know all of that as a medical student, but he learned much that moved the world closer to that understanding.

When Warburg studied embryonic growth as a medical student, he noted fast, uncontrolled growth of cells, as we would expect of embryos. Later, he compared cancer growth to this fast growth. However, whereas embryos used six times the oxygen of normal cells in their energy metabolism, cancer would default to anaerobic growth (that is growth that occurs without oxygen).

The preferred mechanism of cancer growth is fermentation. This is a very inefficient way of living and growing, and a feature that is very important for us to note, because it is cancer's Achilles' heel, and the key to our strength against it. Fermentation is inefficient because it produces only 2 units of energy (ATP) per energy cycle (a metabolic stroll through the citric acid cycle, which is our basic biochemical engine, or at least a large part of it, and which is a bit too detailed for our discussion here).

Whereas our normal cells use aerobic metabolism, a highly efficient mechanism, which produces 38 ATP per cycle, cancer is only about 5% as productive. So it produces only 2 ATP per cycle. Even when cancer exists in an oxygen-rich environment, it defaults or seems to prefer, the inefficient fermentation.

So what is the nature of an inefficient system? One might even say, to study cancer, let's study this particular form of incompetence.

An inefficient machine consumes lots of fuel and produces little output. Warburg observed consumption of glucose in cancer, with relatively little output of ATP. This is known as the Warburg Effect. It is an effect that normal cells do not exhibit. In the presence of oxygen, normal cells do not ferment, but cancer cells do. Despite an oxygen-rich or oxygen-poor environment, cancer cells ferment as if oxygen were not present, and as in other fermentation systems, cancer cells produce a lot of lactic acid.

In fact, there is a principle in chemistry and biochemistry that if you want to stop a particular chemical process, you add a lot of the end-product to the system. In this case, since lactic acid is the result of fermentation in general, including when we pickle cucumbers in the kitchen, it has been proposed to urge the consumption of fermented foods to cancer patients, in order to discourage the cancer machine from using the lactic-acid producing mechanism that it favors. In essence, a feedback inhibition, or negative feedback loop.

There is another thing that Warburg learned from cancer, and that is this: Normal cells, as mentioned above, will not ferment in the presence of oxygen. However, in less than ideal circumstances, say anaerobic conditions in muscles, after strenuous exertion, the fermentative production of lactic acid will occur. So this begs the question: If normal cells will only ferment as last resort, and only as a back-up, inefficient, poor-choice energy system, then is the following possible? Is it possible that cancer cells are originally normal cells that lost their ability to metabolize normally, and that this loss made them default permanently to the less efficient system of fermentation?

And if that is the case, then it raises a really interesting question: What exactly was it that happened to the cell to damage it so that it became cancerous? And it gets even more interesting, when the conventionally accepted answer to the question, that is DNA damage, is not adequate or true. That is, genetic damage did not create the cancer cell. So what did?

This question was destined to be lost to distraction, due to a very compelling event occurring in 1953. Molecular biologists James Watson of the US and Francis Crick of England, announced that they had discovered the form of the molecule at the core of life: the double-helix (twisting ladder) DNA molecule. Their discovery was so dazzling, because of the beauty of the form and because every rung of the ladder was found to code for instructions for everything from eye color to height to predilection for certain diseases, across all plant and animal species. The universally applicable finding was so impressive that other scientists, who had contributed much to the discovery, got kicked down off that ladder on the rise of the much-celebrated Watson and Crick.

Rosalind Franklin was not acknowledged by the pair, but was the first to have discovered the essential structure by her unprecedented quality and precision x-ray diffraction photos of the DNA molecule in January 1953. She had also deduced the double helix structure from mathematical modeling. Only later, in the spring of 1953 did Watson and Crick see Franklin's photograph, without her permission, and published the double helix structure of DNA themselves. [166]

American chemist Linus Pauling had also been in a tight race with the pair, and was close to discovering the molecular structure himself.

Scientists had now found the key to unlocking so many of the mysteries of nature. If we could find genetic programming in this beautiful new but ancient double helix, then we could explain not only inherited traits from one generation to the next, but also we could learn more about hereditary diseases: hemophilia, sickle cell anemia, Tay Sachs. Perhaps all non-infectious diseases really had a genetic origin, perhaps even the biggest mystery: cancer. So in the following decades, medical research investment was off to the races, enthusiastically pursuing genetic explanations for as much of the human condition as possible.

There was one problem with that when it came to cancer, by far the largest target of all of this effort, money and study: Otto Warburg had proven such pursuits of a genetic origin of cancer baseless and unwarranted a full two to three decades before Watson and Crick's famous discovery. But Warburg was neither as famous as he deserved, nor one who had successfully persuaded others to look deeply enough at his work, even after his Nobel Prize. From there on, Warburg, very confident that he was correct, but not so talented at enlightening others, languished in obscurity.

This turn of events effectively postponed for decades the most essential and urgent question regarding cancer, one that could have saved hundreds of thousands of lives: If the cause of cancer is not genetic, then what does cause cancer?

Warburg's experiments with normal cell lines and oxygen deprivation showed this: Take normal cells and deprive them of oxygen, and at first, they will ferment. But if you deprive them of oxygen for hours, even with no other influence, no toxin, no other damage, they will turn cancerous, without returning to normal state. This was the evidence Warburg needed to convince himself that the first carcinogenic event was oxygen deprivation, which disrupted the most basic function of the cell: creating energy for its survival. If you deprive a cell of oxygen, you damage its energy-producing apparatus, now known as the mitochondria, and it is at that point that the cell turns cancerous.

Warburg the Nobel scientist was convinced of this as the fundamental cause of cancer for the rest of his life, yet it would take decades before he was again taken seriously. Warburg had shown how very simple the mechanism of cancer is. Yet much infrastructure and vast fortunes have been built on the notion that cancer is almost hopelessly complex.

Chapter 10

The Problem With Chemotherapy

An increasing number of scientists over recent years have dared to speak up regarding the obsolescence of chemotherapy. Although their hope is usually for adequately targeted gene therapy, which is a dead-end, as explained in Chapter 9, it is an acknowledgment of the unacceptable problems of chemotherapy. I have even heard a number of chemotherapy oncologists admit this in medical conferences in small conversations with their colleagues. Dwight McKee MD is one of the few medical oncologists to go on record with this prediction.[167]

Modern chemotherapy was born in World War II, November 30, 1943, in Bari, Italy. The event was an air attack by the Luftwaffe on Allied warships. Unfortunately, one such ship was stockpiled with an agent of chemical warfare: mustard gas, despite an agreement by both sides not to use war gasses. As Allied servicemen found themselves blown from their ship and into the now contaminated water, an oily residue clung to their skin and clothes. Over the next few days, following rescue from the cold water, they complained of burning skin and blindness. One thousand Allied servicemen lost their lives from this exposure.

Over the next few days after the attack it was discovered that another effect of this gas exposure on the men was that their white blood cells were greatly reduced. Later, the same chemical was then given deliberately and experimentally to lymphoma and leukemia patients, and it was discovered that their cancer burden regressed considerably. This discovery was especially exciting, because conventional medicine had not yet offered any effective treatment at all for any cancer, except for radical surgery and radiation. Neither of those was applicable to such an elusive and scattered blood disease, such as the leukemias. So here was something that appeared to be a viable and promising alternative.

But the excitement was short-lived, because the cancer regression only lasted weeks. The nitrogen mustard in mustard gas attacks DNA, which greatly inhibits cell reproduction.

However, and this is the problem with chemotherapy generally, cells mutate, and are all too soon resistant to the chemotherapy drug that they were exposed to. So the cancer grows once more. But this time, the cancer is a bit less vulnerable. The cancer has seen its attacker and endured and in some non-conscious way (of course), has "learned" from it. I tell my patients that it is a similar situation to taking too little of an antibiotic. By teasing bacteria with too little of an antibiotic, or too-short dosing, you have trained it to become stronger and more resistant. This is obviously not a desirable situation when managing infectious disease. Why then should we allow cancer to learn and fortify itself from our mistakes?

An equally serious problem is that anti-DNA strategies of cancer treatment inevitably hurt the entire body. With conventional dosing of chemotherapy, initially, nausea and vomiting wrack the body. All of the cells of the blood: red and white blood cells and platelets drop to dangerous levels. The GI tract from mouth to anus becomes excoriated with scattered bleeding, as this normally quickly reproducing tissue is stopped from producing more tissue. Finally, after a few weeks the hair cannot make new cells, and the already produced hair falls out.

Much has been made of this loss of hair as being the only horrifying effect of chemotherapy, yet in essence a merely cosmetic inconvenience. However, if you see such drastic destruction as this overall alopecia – no head hair, no eyebrows or eyelashes, and all the way down - on the surface of the body, what kind of destruction do you suppose is taking hold on the inside? Given these devastating effects, is it really any surprise that an agent of war, a chemical poison, was the first chemotherapy agent used?

Later in 1947, methotrexate was developed. Having learned from the temporary remission, relapse and then ultimate failure of the nitrogen mustard in leukemia, scientist Sidney Farber looked for a way to interfere with folic acid use or uptake by the body. Folic acid was necessary for proper DNA function and normal cell replication. Farber wanted a molecule that looked a little like folic acid by the body, enough to be attempted in use by the cells. However, what he mostly wanted was a molecule that would gum up the works, a Trojan horse into a cell. Methotrexate was similar enough to folic acid to be accepted by all the necessary receptor sites, but not similar enough to function adequately as folic acid. Therefore, like the mustard gas, it stopped cell division, and it led to the same devastating effects, with only temporary remission from leukemia.

In 1951, 6-mercaptopurine (6-MP) developed by scientist Gertrude Elion, performed a similar function. As with the two predecessor drugs, remission could be achieved, but only for weeks.

With these three, however, Sidney Farber's goal of amassing an arsenal of multiple chemotherapy drugs was beginning to be realized. That is, Farber had written of inspiration from recent productive developments in antibiotics. A strength of the new arsenal of antibiotics was to have multiple weapons with which to defeat a multi-faceted problem: bacterial resilience. The thinking was that when one antibiotic weakens a bacterium, the next one in a therapeutic series may be likelier to finish the job.

Farber dreamt of a similar arsenal for chemotherapy, enough weapons to be able to eliminate cancer for good. Or at least an ability to switch from one agent to another in the face of resilient cancer growth.

As it turned out, this was later achieved in an area that Farber never thought of looking: the natural world. However, Otto Warburg, who had figured out the nature of cancer over a decade earlier, would likely not have been terribly surprised.

In 1957, two colleagues, Emil Frei and Emil Freireich, were able to realize Farber's goal of combining chemotherapy drugs for more intense impact. Methotrexate and 6-MP were each quite harsh drugs alone. Now in combination, they were so toxic as to bring cancer patients, in this case, children with leukemia, to the brink of death. However, that toxicity also was somewhat effective against the cancer. Remission rose from less than 20% to 45%.[168]

But the price paid for that increase was morally reprehensible: a slow poisoning of children compounding the misery of their already devastating disease. How could their doctors put them through such torture?

Oncologist Max Wintrope of the National Cancer Institute Hospital observed that "These drugs cause more harm than good, because they just prolong the agony. The patients all die anyway." [169] In this bleak environment, the goal was to rid the body of every single cancer cell, in the belief that even one such cell remaining in the body could bring a return of the cancer throughout the body.

Yet the combinations of chemotherapy drugs multiplied, with Freireich's strategy of combining drugs of different types of toxicity, so that a child with leukemia was not attacked so harshly in one particular organ system, but rather with the misery spread throughout the body.

In the 1960's chemotherapy and the field of oncology generally was new, with the first of that field including Frei, Freireich and Vincent DeVita, a cardiologist who joined them in 1963. At the time, they were very much outsiders in the medical field, viewed askance and skeptically by their colleagues who disapproved of the severe toxicity of chemotherapy. Yet each time a cocktail of chemo drugs was given to the children with leukemia, their leukemia at first abated and then came back, usually to the brain, where it was not so accessible to any known treatment, and gradually the patients of the three researchers died of recurrent leukemia. However, by the end of the sixties, with even larger combinations of drugs and targeted to the neurological system, where the leukemic cells were sequestered, children with leukemia were finally going into remission.

Thus chemotherapy entered its long heyday. It seemed that with appropriate combinations of drugs, childhood leukemia could be put into remission. The zeitgeist in the early 1970's was, more than anything else, confidence. A man could walk on the moon. And finally, cancer, one of the most devastating diseases in human history, was being held at bay by pharmaceutical innovation. The budget for drug development at the National Cancer Institute grew to $ 68 million[170] and vetted 40,000 drugs every year. The standard mechanism for the drugs was the same every time: tangling DNA into an unworkable knot, so that cell reproduction was prevented. This stopped all growth, including cancer, and led to the familiar side effects of hair loss and GI tract excoriation, as well as damage to major organs.

James Watson, co-discoverer of the DNA double-helix, and physician/author Eric Topol spoke out against the indiscriminate destructive forces of the chemotherapy regimens, which held the patients on the edge of life and death. He and many others questioned the ethics of delivering the patient to the brink of death, in order to pound the cancer as hard as possible. As a result, Watson was quickly sidelined from those front lines, getting kicked off the advisory board of the National Cancer Institute.

But despite the criticism, NCI's position grew bolder. Instead of only targeting leukemia and other blood dyscrasias, NCI pushed for also using the toxic cocktails with solid tumors, which accounted for the majority of cancer deaths by far.

When the results of all this intervention were finally tallied by statisticians in the mid-1980's the numbers were bleak. Death by cancer had actually increased by 9%. Then more bad news surfaced by the 1990's regarding the survivors. Those treated for Hodgkins lymphoma were 18 times more likely to later develop secondary cancers, and 75 times as likely to develop breast cancer as patients never treated for lymphoma.

This disappointing news renewed calls among the public and the scientific community for more precisely targeted therapies, chemotherapy that could be more of a 'magic bullet.'

That particular prescription was expected by all to be filled by conventional medicine. It wasn't. It is beginning to be filled by natural medicine, as we will see in Part Two.

Chapter 11

How Did Most Doctors Get Trapped Into Disease Management Rather Than Health Counseling?

Probably the overriding mistake that doctors make is to succumb to ill-advised capitulation to pressure from others. Ours is likely the worst profession for being constantly scrutinized for revealing anything short of perfect behavior, with a tribunal in place (the medical board) that would be only too happy to temporarily or permanently, take away a license to practice medicine, in order to show their state's governor and the public that they are tough on bad doctors, and if not by finding a real bad doctor, at least by scapegoating and railroading a random one once in a while.

Thus, physicians endure unbearable pressure to always be perfect, with the gravest consequences for our mistakes. Those who work under the insurance paradigm suffer from ever more unreasonable and voluminous demands by an insurance industry that would prefer to create unreasonable amounts of work for a doctor than to pay on a patient's claim.

For this reason, one of the most fundamental lessons of a conventional medical curriculum – of which I completed the first two years – the entire academic portion - before transferring to naturopathic medical school, was the following: CYA. As this may be more politely translated: Remain sure, at all times, that you cannot be blamed for anything – not by the patient, not by the even more demanding family of the patient, and not by the institution of your employment, and not by – heaven forbid - the regulatory authorities, aka the medical board. This has led to an enormous excess of imaging and blood labs and other labs. It has led to medical doctors charting that they performed physical exams that their patients are certain that they did not do, that they did not even have time to do, in the very abbreviated – in fact, ridiculously short – time allotted by insurance companies for the office consult. (Medicare has even said that they will no longer reimburse for consults requested by Medicare patients, because the only legitimate consultations are those requested by other physicians![171]) So much for the S (patient's report of condition) and P (doctor's plan or instructions discussed with the patient) of the traditionally formatted chart note or "SOAP note." [*] The word "doctor" comes from the Latin 'docere' meaning *to teach*. So much for the historic role of the doctor's counsel to the patient in the Medicare model!

Some of the excessive procedures that doctors are expected to do are an enormous number of blood labs. The fear is that one would miss something if one did

---

[*] The medical chart note is organized as a "SOAP note" – Subjective, for patient's report; Objective, for physician's observations, physical exams, labs, imaging; Assessment, for the diagnosis; and Plan, for the treatment plan.

not test every conceivable lab that could remotely be guessed to be useful to a patient. Hence, a person with rosacea – a benign and chronic redness of the skin – gets a full work-up for lupus, with expensive and exotic blood labs to rule in or out lupus, which is a more serious and much rarer disease than rosacea. The common cold and cough is pronounced to be bronchitis on a slow day at the primary care clinic, with full work-up and chest x-ray.

Likewise, cancer patients and their families, worried sick over the up-to-date results of what's happening with the cancer, tend to demand whatever information can be had, and this is perfectly reasonable and understandable on their part. Blood labs are quick, easy, cheap and convenient.

However, there is one problem: With cancer, blood labs are useless, unless cancer is at a very late stage, and then they will confirm what everybody can see, that the person is in late stage cancer.

When blood labs are done earlier, the results have been very haphazard and inaccurate with regard to patients' conditions. For example, the blood lab that is allegedly indicative of ovarian cancer, CA-125, is so notoriously inaccurate, that it has a 30% false positive and a 30% false negative! [172] That means for any set of 3 women who imagine themselves to be in okay health, one of them will have a positive CA-125.

I will personally never forget an ovarian cancer patient of mine, a RN just several weeks older than me, trained in the medical-doctor-knows-everything paradigm, and even after having my intravenous nutrient treatments for her cancer plus surgery had

154

eliminated her entire tumor burden, and she was confirmed tumor-free for several months, which was a successful outcome for such a dire cancer, and her cancer had been gone all of that time, and she had no physical complaints, she was doomed for the following reason. The MD told her that her CA-125 blood lab was a little high, and that she would have to do chemotherapy. As I say, this is the lab that is perhaps most notoriously flawed of all of the cancer blood labs, which are all very unreliable, for a reason that I will explain below. Anyway, let's call this patient Brenda. Brenda the RN with ovarian cancer, who had zero tumor burden, told me that her MD insisted that she would have to have chemotherapy to bring that CA-125 number down. A number that I knew to be meaningless, but failed to communicate that to the patient, regardless of my many exhortations.

I said to her, "But that chemotherapy could kill you. Are you sure you want to do that? You realize that your PET was clear and you have no tumor burden. We could go over your recent PET/CT again."

She said that she had to do as her chemotherapy oncologist instructed. So with my respectful and regretful acquiescence, or rather despite my protests, she started chemotherapy treatments for the first time, thinking she would be able to handle it.

Guess what: Four rounds of chemotherapy later, she was dead. Alive and well with no tumor burden, and then in several weeks, dead with no tumor burden. As we like to say in the US, what's wrong with this picture? A woman who worked out regularly at her gym, was on her feet and walking all day in the hospital where she worked, she was chemically poisoned, although her cancer had never come back.

What is the lesson from this? What can we do differently in the future that cancer patients may avoid Brenda's fate? Well, not deifying a medical doctor and not consenting to terrible medical advice is a start. But also, patients need to be informed about the fallibility of the blood labs, so that they don't try to read their fate on such a bogus Ouija board as that.

In medicine, we talk about the sensitivity of a test. That is the ability to detect all the people who are sick. Then we also look at the specificity of a test. That is the ability to pronounce healthy all those who are not sick.

In medicine, sensitivity is the ability to diagnose those with a disease state. 100% sensitivity finds all persons with disease in the examined population. A laboratory test that finds half of the diseased individuals has 50% sensitivity.

Similarly, specificity finds the non-affected or healthy individuals in the examined population. 100% specificity correctly identifies all of the unaffected individuals in a given population. Poor specificity occurs when many of the healthy people are assumed to be diseased.

Natural cancer doctors also fall for labs that are fairly useless, and many popular blood and urine labs have been touted over the years, until a broad consensus notices that patient results don't track with the labs. Then that lab also falls from favor, until another is touted as the definitive story.

A popular lab as of this writing – because there is always a flavor of the month lab being touted - was described to me by a doctor as the latest and greatest in cancer diagnosis. I asked how many patients he had used the lab with: 50. And how many patients' cancers tracked with that lab? 3 or 4. Hmmm. So far, not at all impressive. Could he please describe his best case where the lab tracked with the cancer as expected? Well, the lab went in one direction and the patient's tumor burden increased – the opposite of the predicted direction. Well, that was not a convincing argument to me.

Cancer blood labs are all bad because of one overriding feature of cancer: It is parasitic in nature. Just as an epiphyte sucking life from a tree, it takes from the body, and does not give, except for waste. Those waste products are not identifiably specific to cancer. It does not donate anything recognizable, anything that is peculiar to cancer alone, and that can be measured, to the best of my knowledge and experience.

Mistake #1 that doctors make: Over-reliance and faith in "cancer marker" blood labs of extremely poor quality. Face it, doctors: the state-of-the-art of those labs is abysmal. Generations from now, maybe good quality, reliable cancer marker labs will be available. Maybe there is something that at least some cancers put into the blood that are identifiable as such. That particular technology is not accessible in our time. Face it, and make do without it, before you kill any more patients with bogus data and bad advice.

*   *   *

The next major mistake doctors make is by far the biggest, although when patients make this mistake – and most of them do – the patients are the bigger victims.

Let's begin with a brief history of the massive and monopolistic pharmaceutical industry. It wasn't always so big.

Benjamin Rush, MD, a signer of the Declaration of Independence, had warned to the Continental Congress, "The Constitution of this Republic should make special provision for medical freedom. Unless we put medical freedom into the Constitution, the time will come when medicine will organize into an undercover dictatorship and force people who want doctors and treatment of their own choice to submit to only what the dictating outfit offers."[173] Very unfortunately, Dr. Rush's contemporaries did not appreciate the wisdom of his advice, and medical freedom is still not explicitly recognized in the US, except for in the use of Informed Consent. Vaccination is presented as mandatory by pediatricians and by many schools, unfortunately. Chemotherapy is offered to cancer patients as the only solution.

But it would be more than a century till Dr. Rush's sage prophecy and advice became thoroughly fulfilled. At the turn of the century 1900, Americans relied mostly on herbs and certain foods for their medicine. This was not simply because Hippocrates had said millennia earlier: "Let your medicine be your food, and your food be your medicine." Rather, that was simply what was known, familiar, available, and fairly unchallenged by other entities.

About that time, the Rockefeller and Carnegie families perceived that their petrochemical investments could be most richly rewarded if products of that industry could begin to be perceived as medicine.

On the face of it, this was a truly absurd idea: We had inherited the bodies of our recent and distant ancestors, who had relied entirely on plants and animals for both medicine and food. To now shift to a petrochemical source for medicine was as silly as trying to make a vegetarian animal such as a rabbit eat meat. That is, there was simply no inherited precedent for it. It couldn't work, unless . . .

The challenge for Rockefeller and Carnegie was to sell their petrochemical nostrums on an uninterested public and an unconvinced medical profession. They had found that if they manipulated substances a bit, they could have some effect in the body, if only causing new symptoms to overwhelm old symptoms.

So Abraham Flexner, an educator, not in medicine, was sent in to begin the overhaul. In 1910, the Flexner report condemned all but two of the many homeopathic, osteopathic, naturopathic and chiropractic schools in the US, while praising the conventional medical schools. This was quite an upheaval, a fork in the road where the US is still on the path Flexner forged. The natural medical practitioners did not have their own governing boards, and were more easy prey for the Rockefeller / Carnegie agenda. The MDs, those still using silver and other toxic substances as "medication," survived the purge with their medical schools intact and strengthened. Most medical schools were shuttered. Those that remained were models for newer medical schools using the Rockefeller / Carnegie / AMA / Johns Hopkins laboratory model of making substances that could be patented and sold as remedies.

It also had the effect of winnowing the diversity of medical practitioners to simply the MDs. The Flexner report was praised by its sympathizers for eliminating schools with whose pedagogy they disagreed, and on the grounds that the purge took competition away from the medical doctors, and allowed the MDs to begin their near monopoly of human health. Coincidentally, it was the very medical schools who were not doing enough to purvey the new petrochemical drugs to satisfy the needs of the new drug industry which found themselves shuttered by Flexner's dictates.

So the relatively few physicians who could still legally practice medicine evolved into an elite, and much of the remnants and trappings of the dictatorial stance of the prescribing physician is still in place, ever since the Flexner Report eliminated a number of medical professions, leaving a demand-side economy for medical providers, with too few, and much sought-after, doctors. By 1925, over 10,000 herbalists went out of business, and over 1,500 chiropractors would be prosecuted for practicing quackery.[174] However, because the new pharmaceuticals were unpopular, they were purveyed in a supply-side economy.

In an impossible bind, the chiropractors were prosecuted for practicing medicine without a license, but in that time, there had not existed any specifically chiropractic board, as there is today, to have granted to them such a license.

Interestingly, the terms "quack" and "quackery," which are usually applied sloppily to whomever the speaker disdains, are derived from the German *Quacksilber*, which means mercury - a substance used in the drug tradition, certainly not in the herbalist or naturopathic or chiropractic tradition.

Nevertheless, having no valid dispute with natural doctors, the new advocates of the profession, headed by Morris Fishbein of the AMA, resorted to labelling the natural practitioners with the term "quack." The new medical profession wallowed in hypocrisy: for-profit scams, corruption amongst a closed circle of elites became the norm. Writer Ty Bollinger describes the post-Flexner period as having taken the vibrant color wheel that was medicine in the US and chopped out all colors except a dull uniform gray. As predicted by Dr. Rush, as quoted at the top of Chapter One, medicine was congealing quickly into an "outfit" closed to outsiders, and offering its wares as the public's only option.

Another effect, more pertinent to individual physicians up to this day, was the removal of compounding from practicing physicians, with a division of labor that removed other physicians to laboratories to come up with the new drugs. Practicing physicians were expected to simply apply those unfamiliar substances to the patients before them. As one might expect, this did not go over well in the clinical setting. For the first time, the treating doctor was expected to be no more than a drug pusher of what the more respected and better compensated research doctors had come up with in the laboratory – the increasingly expensive patented nostrums that we see so heavily advertised in our time. Clinicians chafed at the role, and it was certainly fought in court repeatedly.

And then, having enough rope, the AMA and the medical profession as a whole committed excesses to the point of trouble. The work of Dr. Royal Raymond Rife, inventor of the machine of his name, as well as the Hoxsey Formula and use of it were nearly destroyed by the medical pharmaceutical cabal, despite much documented success of each against cancer and a number of other diseases.

The Fitzgerald Report, written by Benedict Fitzgerald, an investigator for the Interstate Commerce Commission, and published in the *Congressional Record* in 1953, finally took the monopoly to task. Fitzgerald was hired by Congressman Charles Tobey, after Tobey's son was cured of an allegedly fatal cancer, using only natural treatments.

The Fitzgerald Report was damning indeed: It charged the AMA with foul play: racketeering and conspiracy to suppress and withhold natural treatments and cures for especially cancer. Identifying conspiratorial acts committed in multiple US states, Fitzgerald wrote: "Behind and over all this [racketeering] is the weirdest conglomeration of corrupt motives, intrigue, selfishness, jealousy, obstruction and conspiracy that I have ever seen."[175]

Although the AMA and the American Cancer Society had insisted that the only cures for cancer were radiation and surgery, Fitzgerald listed in his Report the names and addresses of patients who were found by pathological reports to be cured of their cancers after treatment at the Hoxsey clinics, and without any of the conventional treatments.[176] Hoxsey treatment involves a synergy of herbs and nutrients primarily.

Fitzgerald labeled the actions of the American Medical Association and American Cancer Association as "the greatest hoax of our time" regarding their attacks on alternative cancer therapies. He regarded them as a cartel existing in order to protect their monopolies of radiation and surgery as the exclusive treatments for cancer. He was perhaps the first well-known figure to make cogent and damning arguments against the abusive medical monopolists, such as the following:

> We should determine whether existing agencies, both public and private, are engaged and have pursued a policy of harassment, ridicule, slander and libelous attacks on others sincerely engaged in stamping out this curse [cancer] of mankind. Have medical associations through their officers, agents, servants and employees engaged in this practice?
>
> Public and private funds have been thrown about like confetti at a county fair to close up and destroy clinics, hospitals and scientific research laboratories which do not conform to the viewpoint of medical associations.
>
> How long will the American people take this? It is but another manifestation of power and privilege of a few at the expense of the many.

But it was later that Fitzgerald's efforts were vindicated. An 11-year court battle begun by Chester Wilk, DC, a doctor of chiropractic, took the AMA to task for anti-competitive actions, in their relentless defamation of the chiropractic profession, and attempts to eliminate that profession altogether. After a long antitrust battle, US District Judge Susan Getzendanner filed her scathing ruling that the AMA, the American College of Radiology and the American College of Surgeons were guilty of violating the Sherman Antitrust Act.[177] This Act is an inviolable act of Congress, in which prison time and fines in the millions of dollars are mandated for violators.[178] The AMA and its co-defendants were not in that category, and therefore escaped the worst punishments.

The AMA, in the same ruling, also had to answer for its actions against its own members, medical doctors who had referred to chiropractors. Finally, in this ruling, the worst of the medical profession's anti-competitive behavior was called to task.

Even given that confrontational and courageous history, in our times, there is so very much more work still to do to dismantle the near monopoly, and near stranglehold, of conventional medicine on human health. As cited in the beginning of this book, the major media in the United States receives 70% of its revenue, in non-election years, from Pharma. Is it any wonder then that you never hear the words "chiropractor," "naturopathic physician," "herbalist" or "acupuncturist" in the mainstream media? Pharma has purchased its monopoly of the public conversation, just as it has purchased Congress. There are more Pharma lobbyists in Congress than for any other industry.[179]

Worse yet, several generations of Americans, since the federal Food, Drug and Cosmetic Act of 1938, [180] have been persuaded by bombardment with drugs and drug ads and drug culture for everything from a Tylenol to cool a fever, to statin drugs to suppress the non-existent problem of robust serum cholesterol. Previous generations knew that fever is a valuable innate tool that we have to resolve acute contagious illness, even without the germ theory. They knew that chronic pain is not a necessary accompaniment to old age, and they knew that proper movement, as taught by traditional osteopaths and chiropractors, is a far more effective and long-lasting solution to pain than is an aspirin tablet. But decades of Pharma indoctrination has got people actually believing that human health is better achieved with a molecule that the human body is not repaired by, and often distracts from our original symptom with new side effects – as if that were more effective and preferable to the movement, the nutrients, the herbs with which our species has spent millenia in close association.

With such a complete shut-out of dissent from the pharmaceutical model in American culture, American politics and American lifestyle, how have Americans imagined any challenge at all to a pharmaceutical lifestyle?

It may be that all we have on our side is common sense: the wisdom that we human beings, descended from and physically similar to earlier human beings, clearly have a congenital, ongoing need for a full-range of nutrients, and that there is no congenital need for isolated, manufactured synthetic molecules such as pharmaceuticals.

What is especially needed to mount an effective challenge to the pharmaceutical model of health is this, no more or less than this: A critical mass of individuals in each community and social stratum and workplace who exemplify the healthier lifestyle by choices in whole, natural foods, increased movement in the form of exercise, and avoidance of pharmaceuticals and other toxins. Only in this way, will those who still only imagine a couch-potato / junk food / drug-every-symptom lifestyle – only then will they begin to notice that there is a better, far more satisfactory and more comfortable and much more pleasant way of living.

Chapter 12

Four major dietary mistakes made by most cancer patients

Given a disease as difficult as cancer, as one might imagine, the choices made by a cancer patient have tremendous impact on the course of the disease, the ease or difficulty of regaining health, indeed the very survival of the individual.

This is all the more true in an outpatient setting. Whereas a hospitalized patient, or one under a highly toxic regimen, has the daily routine arranged by others, the ambulatory outpatient, in contrast, decides for themselves such routine events as diet and exercise and sleep habits.

One of the most common mistakes cancer patients make is to take any of those for granted, or without careful consideration among available choices.

In the 21st century developed world, food choices are more varied than ever before in human history, and people even in the same family can eat vastly differently from each other if they so choose. In Chapters 7 and 8 we showed how food choices can make life or death difference in cancer. We have found in our clinical practice that many dietary differences among cancer patients that create a flutter on the internet are of very little consequence. On the other hand, our clinic has conducted the longest and largest study to date of sugar consumption in cancer patients, and found an overwhelming difference in remission and survival between the sugar eaters and the sugar avoiders. See Chapter 8.

However simple this concept is, and however well-documented in the medical literature going back almost a century, people still seek out and travel long distances to our clinic with considerable unease and confusion regarding the role of sugars in cancer growth and progression.

Most cancer patients arrive saying that they have had a history of being a "sweet tooth." This seems to be especially true for the pancreatic cancer patients, which should be easily understood when we consider one of the primary roles of the pancreas – one of the main reasons we even *have* a pancreas, is to regulate the amounts and distribution of sugar in the blood. Therefore, the pancreas has likely suffered some damage or at least extreme conditions by the time the individual receives a diagnosis of pancreatic cancer.

But it is not only pancreatic cancer patients who enter our clinic with confusion over the role of sugar in cancer or what even constitutes "sugar." Not by a long shot. Almost everyone asks in their first or second consult if it is alright to have honey or maple syrup or alcohol sugars. This is even after the first day, in which the individualized protocol we recommend – which is quite varied from one patient to the next - generally includes identical, one-size-fits-all boilerplate language of the following form: "It is essential to avoid sweeteners except for stevia." This is bold, underlined and highlighted in yellow. Yet the most frequent question that we get from patients is what other sweeteners may be acceptable besides stevia.

It's not that our patients have trouble comprehending what we ask. Far from it; they have considered their options carefully, and have carefully and intelligently made the best and most survivable decision possible in coming to our clinic, I sincerely believe, and as we have amply demonstrated in Chapter 7.

Rather, the problem is that sugar – like tobacco or alcohol – is a hard habit to kick, and giving it up all at once is a bracing and unpleasant prospect for many of our newcomers. They are looking for a way to have their cake and eat it too. Who can blame them, given the fond memories they've acquired throughout their lives of enjoying special occasions with our most globally acceptable social lubricant – desserts, sweets, soda and candy? Yet, this is the very thing I ask them to give up – with the lame apology that I am the Grinch that stole the Christmas cookies.

I consider it my responsibility to offer satisfactory substitutes whenever I can, for the sweeteners that I've asked my patients to forgo. In our IV rooms, we have various stevia recipes, for such treats as apple pie or frozen coconut/carob cubes and a number of others. Some of them will most dearly miss sweetener in their coffee. For others, the delectable treat is ice cream, and for others it is chocolate. In each case, I make some suggestions until we discuss something palatable that can be made without high glycemic sweeteners. For ice cream, we discuss different fruits that can be added to heavy cream in a blender, to approximate the flavor and texture of ice cream. For chocolate, I recommend 85% cocoa content or higher, one or two small squares per day, in order to try to keep the sugar intake at 3 grams or less. In each case, over the course of our regular consults, patients usually want to discuss food choices and dessert strategies more than any other single topic.

Also, I consider it my responsibility to eat only as I ask my patients to eat. Therefore, I have no sweets at all in my diet, except those sweetened with stevia, and my family follows the same diet, regardless of holidays or birthdays. (We know how to make some very nice holiday cookies with stevia and a stevia pumpkin pie on Thanksgiving, etc.) When I make apple pie at home, I actually don't add any sweetener at all. I simply put apple slices, cinnamon, butter, coconut oil and flour into an unsweetened pie crust, bake at 40 minutes, and that seems to be a nice treat.

Stevia also unfortunately does not grow with an instructional pamphlet attached to the stem, though it would likely be a lot more popular if that were a feature of the plant. The uninitiated assume that stevia will be less sweet than sugar, when in fact it is many times sweeter, hundreds of times more perceptibly sweet, in fact, in a volume-by-volume comparison. Therefore, those trying stevia for the first time often make the mistake of putting a teaspoonful or so in a cup of coffee or other drink, and then nearly gagging at the very unpalatable result. In fact, it takes anywhere from 7 to

12 *drops* only to sweeten a drink to satisfaction.

I hear more than any other single protest, "I tried stevia, and I don't like it." My response is, "That's likely because you had too much. Try this glass of lemonade: Squeeze ¼ lemon into a glass of water, and add 8 drops only of liquid stevia. Then you may want to add one or two more drops. I think you will find it to be far more pleasant than what you had before." It seems a majority of patients had such a jarring experience with their first encounter with stevia that they don't want to try the lemonade, and simply choose to give up all sweets. Fortunately, this abstinence is usually successful at our clinic, because the patients understand that the stakes are quite high. If they had met with the hundreds of patients we have met with over the last decade, and had gotten to know the sweet-eaters who then died of cancer, they would know that the stakes are indeed quite a bit higher than they had imagined.

Thus we plug along on a daily basis, addressing our patients' sugar nostalgia and anxiety on recipe-by-recipe basis, attempting to forge some common ground of acceptability, negotiating away this and urging that, hoping that they will each find some comfort and diligence in pursuing the new diet.

Those who have made the mistake of not following the recommendation to eliminate sweeteners have more often than not (64% of the time in fact, as seen in Chapter 8) broken our hearts, and we have sent sympathy cards to their bereaved families.

In 2016, two of the lucky ones, survivors, came back at the same time to our clinic with cancer recurrence.

One was extroverted and the other was quiet by nature. They had each given up sweets, had a few months of our IV nutrient treatments for breast cancer and lymphoma respectively, and had gone into remission a few years earlier, and stayed in remission during those years. Then over time away from us, each began to eat sweets again. The extroverted patient recently told all fellow patients who would listen: "Don't do what I did. I began to eat sugar again, and my cancer came back." As might be imagined, her first-hand account was far more persuasive to the other patients than anything that I might say, although I used many more words and hours to say it. Certainly, there are a number of cancer survivors already who now owe their lives in part to her very timely warning.

Mistake Number 1: Continuing to eat sweets after a cancer diagnosis. This, in our experience, is an even more likely cause of cancer-related death than chemotherapy or continued smoking. See Chapter 8.

*   *   *

There is another enormously common mistake that cancer patients make:

Like much of the rest of the western hemisphere, cancer patients have been urged by the zeitgeist at large to become vegetarian for better health. On being diagnosed with cancer, and being forced to stare at the specter of one's own mortality, the time seems urgent to finally follow the widely broadcast advice to become vegetarian or vegan. However, an extraordinarily high number of cancer patients had chosen this path long before diagnosis, and are then dismayed when they

172

find themselves with cancer after making "healthier" choices than most of their peers and loved ones.

Now I will readily acknowledge that a vegetarian diet may well be a preferable choice for a huge portion of the world's population, varying considerably from say parts of India to say for example the Inuit, perhaps each of them being near the extremes on that particular dichotomy of vegan/vegetarian to omnivore to carnivore, among all human populations. Most of the rest of us throughout the world fall somewhere in between those polar opposites on the vegan-vegetarian-omnivore-carnivore continuum.

I will also acknowledge that a vegan or vegetarian diet is much kinder to the planet and its domesticated animal inhabitants than any alternative. A plant-based diet is also far more efficient since it takes over two pounds of plant material and over a thousand gallons of water to make one pound of beef,[181] and it takes only dozens or hundreds of gallons of water to make one pound of plant material.[182] With the earth's still accelerating increase in human inhabitants on our Malthusian curve toward "population explosion," and the domesticated animals that feed us, these numbers must be considered with increasing urgency globally in order to feed us all.

However, when it comes to an individual who, at this relatively brief period of life, is suffering with cancer, such considerations must be put aside.

Much as I think that people without cancer could reasonably consider a vegetarian diet, those with cancer cannot afford such a luxury. The reason is that ultimately, even the best quality carbohydrates break down and metabolize to a greater amount of sugar/glucose in the blood than the two dietary alternatives: fat and protein.

In fact, that's all we get. Regardless of the lovely smorgasbord available in 21st century supermarkets, if you look at it all in its most basic form, we have three types of food: carbohydrates, proteins and fats.

Considering that carbohydrates, even those of the highest quality, the colorful vegetables, ultimately break down to sugars, we need to adopt the following strategy with cancer patients: Use proteins and especially fats to crowd out, or to displace, carbohydrates in the diet of cancer patients. Of the appetite that remains for carbohydrates, let us default primarily to those of highest quality: the green and yellow vegetables.

I certainly did not invent this strategy. It not only proceeds logically from the findings of Otto Warburg, but such a diet already has a name: the ketogenic diet, as well as its more popular and easier approximation, the paleo diet, which I described and advocated in my 2007 book, <u>Choose Your Foods Like Your Life Depends On Them</u>, a book that was published before the Paleo Diet became popular, with the book of that name published in 2010.[183] However, I certainly was not the first, and won't be the last by any means to advocate such a diet. Every few years somebody writes the latest version of a healthy omnivore's diet. Sally Fallon and Mary Enig's book <u>Nourishing Traditions</u> is highly respected and the most comprehensive work I know with respect to a paleo-type diet.

A strict ketogenic diet is comprised 80% of fat and 20% of a combination of proteins and carbohydrates. As we can imagine, this really leaves no room for a jelly donut or even a spinach salad. Imagine a bacon cheeseburger without a bun. Imagine a cup of heavy cream, with a little coffee added for flavor, a tablespoon of coconut oil and some nuts as a snack. Such a diet is not really the kind of diet that has appealed to the western palate. But there is a far worse problem with it: it is so extreme and restrictive that it is not tenable long-term. Yet the cancer patient needs to survive cancer long-term, and that is the dilemma that must be resolved to their ongoing satisfaction and to their best of health.

Ketogenic diets have been wonderfully helpful in some of the most intractable cancers.[184] [185] Yet despite this very encouraging success, the ketogenic diet is not permanently helpful unless it can be tolerated all the way through to remission. And in my experience, there's the rub. That has been the deal breaker.

Mistake Number 2 then for the cancer patient is abandoning the ketogenic diet with a reckless plunge into the candy store.

I would not go there if I were you. If you want to abandon the ketogenic diet while you still have cancer, I would go paleo. It's more tolerable long-term. People stay on a paleo diet for years and grow very comfortable with it. It will likely be tolerable for you well past evidence of your remission. Then if you want to ease off of that, you can go a little more vegetarian.

If even a Paleo Diet is ultimately too restrictive, then have a Mediterranean Diet. This is primarily composed of vegetables, with substantial olive oil, moderate meats and whole grains. Again, desserts, sweets, sodas, candy are absolutely off-limits, out of the question.

However, I advise you not to adopt the Mediterranean Diet while you have an active cancer. Wait until you are in confirmed remission for at least a year, and then you can transition to the Mediterranean Diet.

But you will never be able to eat sweets again. Period. For life. The same life sentence that I am on and am grateful for, because I always feel well and strong, although I am growing alarmingly old. At least, I find such high numbers alarming. It's okay; before you realize it, you can become comfortable with the Paleo or the Mediterranean lifestyle.

*   *   *

The third mistake is closely related. People often assume that veganism or vegetarianism is a good strategy to adopt during a bout with cancer. It is not, as I have argued above.

A closely related problem is that sprinkled throughout the internet is the very ill-advised suggestion that if eating vegan is good during cancer, then juicing vegetables must be even better. Even worse, one of the oldest, most widely known natural cancer clinics advocate juicing carrots to cancer patients.

This absolutely abysmal suggestion often begins with the self-righteous assertions of non-cancer patients, people who never had cancer, who chose a vegan lifestyle for themselves. 'If I chose to be vegan, you should follow me and be vegan too.'

What a horrible mistake. What horrible tumors we have seen at our clinic, after people followed this bad advice for months and years, until their relentlessly growing tumor finally convinced them they were on the wrong path. How many more deaths and how much worse morbidity will these clinics cause, until they finally realize the horror of what they've done? Anybody who has cancer and is juicing carrots should stop immediately. I say that across the board, regardless of the stage or type of cancer or condition of the individual. Unless a person is so close to death that the only tolerable nourishment is a few sips of carrot juice, then there is no benefit.

Please eat a carrot or two instead.

I will explain why it is such a horrific mistake for a cancer patient to juice vegetables or fruits. A 16-oz glass of freshly pressed carrot juice has 18 grams of sugar. A 16-oz glass of orange juice has 42 grams of sugar.[186] Juicing either fruits or vegetables is a problem for this reason: The fiber in the fruit or vegetable slows down the entry of sugar to the bloodstream, because in the process of early digestion from mouth to stomach, the juice in the fruit or vegetable ends up trickling in at a much slower pace than if you were to drink it. When you drink the juice, there is no such filter, no such rate-limiting process. Therefore, the sugar in that produce enters the bloodstream faster than the pancreas can provide insulin to place the sugar into cells. It is very slightly better to add the pulp back into the juice, and eat that soupy slurry instead, but you still have a dangerously high glycemic assault even in this preparation.

It has been shown that if you eat an apple, you have only a modest rise in blood sugar, with a likewise modest rise in insulin. However, if you take the very same size and type of apple and juice it, your blood sugar rises precipitously, with a likewise high-amplitude disturbance of insulin release, setting your metabolism on an unhelpful roller coaster. Thus, with juicing, a large bolus of glucose in the blood is available suddenly in large amount to a growing, grasping tumor, which thrives on little else but sugar.

Mistake Number 3 is juicing vegetables and fruits. Please don't do that; please eat the whole vegetable or fruit, with limitation on quantity of fruit.

*   *   *

The next mistake is somewhat similar to Mistake Number Two, and it has arisen from misconceptions that have come from certain individuals who do not work with cancer patients. When researchers who work in the laboratory begin to consult with clinicians who work with real people, who happen to have cancer, then I think our understanding of cancer and how to move forward will improve.

But first I must debunk another hypothesis that is making the rounds among those interested in natural treatments for cancer.

Otto Warburg clearly pointed to sugar as the main factor that makes cancer worse. Actually, it is not the *cause* of cancer. That, as Warburg showed, is different, and I will get to that in the next chapter. However, sugar is the fuel that keeps cancer alive, thriving and growing unchecked.

Somehow, it has also been assumed, without basis, that glutamine – which is an amino acid – that is *not* glucose-based, was involved with cancer.

I disagree with that view. Glucose is a sugar, and it fuels cancer growth. Glutamine is not only an amino acid, it is the most common amino acid in the proteins in our food. And it has been the most commonly eaten amino acid throughout human history, including in the great majority of our history when cancer was exceedingly rare. Sugar, in the forms of various sweeteners, is the substance that has sky-rocketed in use just in recent generations, tracking closely in populations with the rapid increase in cancer incidence. Sugar is the fuel for cancer, not glutamine. But the innocence of glutamine is not only established by human history, but also by biochemistry, because it does not contribute to anaerobic fermentation. That is, the substrate for anaerobic fermentation is only sugars, not the amino acids.

Therefore, there are those who advocate, without scientific basis, that cancer patients also avoid proteins, in order to minimize glutamine.

That is terrible advice. Glutamine is not only the most abundant non-essential amino acid. It is consumed in normal tissue more than ten times as much as any other amino acid.[187] Cancer patients need to consume proteins and fats in order to crowd out or to displace carbohydrates from their overall food consumption, and to have the fuel to keep themselves going and thriving and staying active, the urgent necessity of which I will show in Chapter 14, Exercise and Oxygen.

Now there are 3 basic types of foods, as I mentioned before: carbohydrates, proteins and fats. If a cancer patient avoids both carbohydrates and proteins, there is little left to consume but fat. And that is a diet that is hard enough to tolerate with a strict ketogenic diet (80% fat, 20% carbohydrates plus proteins.)

But worse, there are writers who advocate fasting to cancer patients. Sometimes this has the euphemism of "dietary energy reduction." Basically, fasting deprives fuel to everything in the body. The thinking was that cancer is an especially fast-growing tissue, so then fasting would deprive cancer more and more intensely than it would deprive the normal tissue comprising the rest of the body. The justification for this is that cancerous cells deprived of fuel undergo apoptosis rather than necrosis. Apoptosis is the cell death of normal tissue, easier and cleaner for the body to process and dispose of than necrotic tissue.[188]

One author, not a clinician, asks:

"Is it better to kill tumor cells using toxic drugs, as is currently done in the oncology field, or is it better to kill tumor cells using a nontoxic metabolic therapy like [dietary energy restriction]?[189]

I would respond that a poor therapy is not a satisfactory alternative to an abysmal therapy, when successful and tolerable natural therapies exist and are increasingly widely used, as we will see in later chapters.

180

The arguments in favor of fasting for cancer patients are not strong arguments. The strongest argument offered by the above author is that normal healthy volunteers were able to lower their blood glucose when fasting, and because cancer thrives on glucose, we should be able to help starve cancer by semi-starving the patient.[190] That argument is only slightly better than having an appendectomy in order not to have cancer of the appendix, or a double mastectomy, in the hope of avoiding breast cancer – never mind that breast cancer can occur in the remaining tissue close to the chest wall.

Mistake Number 4 is fasting and the avoidance of protein. Do not fast, at least no more than a 12 or 24 hour fast, such as the religious fasts or intermittent fasting, because you will need to eat for the exercise that is absolutely essential to your survival as I will describe in the next chapter. Do not avoid protein for the same reason.

*　　*　　*

There is a growing pile of corpses to whom I could say "I told you so." In fact, I have not been wrong yet about the exact course that each of my patients should pursue. The ones who listened to me have fared the best, except the small minority with already uncontrollable, relentless cancers. Let me please say "I told you so" through this book while you are still alive and still have an opportunity to survive cancer. No corpse can hear me say it, and it wouldn't do any good if they could, and it is far too cruel and useless to say to the surviving loved ones.

There are those who will say that I write too strictly, that I have dared to take on too many of the misconceptions, lies and utterly abysmal advice of my contemporaries in oncology all at once. A more prudent writer would dare to rebel against only one poorly conceived nostrum at a time, without dismissing all bad dogma simultaneously.

To them I say this: The cancer patient sitting in front of me has perhaps a few months to live if they get this wrong, if they do not figure out whether it is my opponents or it is I telling them the truth. They don't have time for those who know nothing but preach loudly to be gently persuaded or for me to delicately hold the chemotherapy oncologists' hands as I guide them to a gradual and painless enlightenment.

Besides, as I established at the beginning of this book, my highest allegiance is to the wellbeing of the cancer patient who has done me the honor of entrusting me with their care, within the confines of the law. I do not apply for membership in any Exclusive Club for Sclerosed Thought, which so many modern clinicians have organized themselves into.

So I will not waste my cancer patients' time. Those who offer bad advice to cancer patients are mere flies buzzing around their numbered meals. They must now stop misguiding people with their bad advice before any more lives are lost as a result.

Part 2

Why cancer is beatable

Chapter 13

What should a cancer patient eat? A sample dietary plan

I have done a fair amount, no, actually, a large amount of complaining about other doctors in this book.

So now I should admit one of my own shortcomings. It's the one that cancer patients complain to me about far more than anything else. It frustrates many of my patients that I recommend certain dietary restrictions and parameters, without doing the constructive work of offering a food plan.

First, I would like to say two or three things in my defense: Different patients come in with different ways of craving sugar: Some want their coffee to be sweet, while others prefer chocolate, and others like ice cream. Therefore, I tailor my one-on-one consults to the expressed needs of the patient in front of me. When I ask them not to eat sugary ice cream, I try to be ready to offer alternative recipes that I have made. The next individual may prefer to hear about my stevia cookie recipe instead.

My second reason for not offering specific food plans is I really don't want to limit the massive supermarket buffet of whole, natural foods to the much smaller number of items that I may happen to think of to put into a food plan.

My third reason is that I am more adventurous in my own diet than I expect of cancer patients. I actually eat raw eggs, barely sautéed chicken livers (perhaps even raw at times!) and raw sushi. For the squeamish and highly germophobic among us, let me now provide the disclaimer that any recommendations below for raw animal products are to be taken with proper prudence, and a grain of salt. Although they would likely taste better with an entire dash of sea salt.

That is, please don't sue me if you acquire salmonella after a raw egg. I take the risk myself, because I fear a relatively short course of salmonella much less than I fear the less than optimal health from forever shunning raw eggs. We should all make our choices with eyes wide open. Please assess your risks with all available information and propaganda, even knowing that lines are very blurry between these two.

The following food plan will still be frustratingly broad to some, but may still possibly address a cancer patient's wish for guidance in at least the beginning of the lifestyle I have asked them to adopt.

Sample weekly food plan

	Breakfast	Lunch	Dinner	Snacks
Sunday	Crustless bacon and cheddar quiche	Caesar salad, with chopped chicken	Butter chicken. Sautéed spinach with garlic, olive oil and sea salt	Macadamia nuts
Monday	Eggnog: Unsweetened coconut milk with raw egg, cinnamon powder and splash of vanilla extract	Left over butter chicken on top of arugula or romaine. Drizzle with olive oil. Dash sea salt.	Salmon, baked and steamed asparagus. Hollandaise sauce for both.	Cashews
Tuesday	Whole avocado with salsa	Leftover salmon and asparagus over dandelion greens	Buffalo or beef chili	Pecans
Wednesday	Eggnog again: Unsweetened coconut milk, cinnamon, raw egg, a little vanilla. Perhaps with raw kefir or raw milk or goat milk if available	Leftover chili on dandelion greens	Almond flour/ coconut flour pizza dough with tomato sauce, sausage, sautéed peppers, mozzarella	Walnuts
Thursday	Whole avocado with salsa	Leftover pizza, and/or kebabs of mozzarella/ cherry tomato/ basil leaves	Eggplant parmesan	Almonds

Friday	Corn thins with cream cheese and pecans	Leftover eggplant parmesan on arugula with olive oil, sea salt	Chicken, celery, onion, carrot stir fry with soy sauce and sesame oil	Peanuts
Saturday	Scrambled eggs with sausage and peppers	Peanut butter and apple slices on corn thins	Buffalo or beef burgers with onion, lettuce, tomato, cheese and leftover sauce from eggplant parmesan	Hazelnuts

Notes:

1) Be sure to make enough food at each dinner, so that you can take leftovers to lunch the next day on top of salad greens. Keep a bottle of olive oil and some sea salt at your work place if possible, in order to add these just before eating.

2) A convenient and non-toxic way to carry lunch to work is to put it into a glass casserole dish with a tight-fitting lid, and into an insulated bag that has a freezer pack in it. Freeze that freezer pack the night before, pop it into the lunch bag, and put your lunch on top of it. This will keep your lunch cool if you don't have access to a refrigerator at work.

3) The reader can probably guess, from a quick glance at this or any other weekly food plan, that the entries are highly interchangeable. Clearly, if dandelion

greens or basil leaves, for example, are not in season at the time, then other raw salad greens will certainly suffice.

4) I have listed 7 different types of nuts, including a botanically questionable nut, really a legume, namely peanuts. I have deliberately written more variety into this list than I would normally have at my own home, in order to make two points:

- Somehow, many cancer patients have gotten the idea (not from me!) that they may eat almonds and no other kind of nut. I wish "experts" who know nothing of nutrition or cancer would immediately stop dispensing advice about the same. Of course, you can eat any edible nuts you like at any time.

- I want to drive home the point that variety is to be emphasized here above all other considerations. Nutrition is a *synergy* of nutrients, a variety of foods. This consideration is paramount in having a healthy diet. So please don't work so hard to exorcise demons out of your diet, other than the sweeteners.

5) I have left out many, many healthy foods, and many recipes, simply because 21

meals per week is the maximum feasible for most of us, and there were only so many suggestions that I could make. My own lack of imagination at breakfast is apparent, and that monotony is part of my unimaginative morning routine. So this diet plan can certainly be improved upon, especially with regard to breakfast.

6) Recipes for quiche, chili, butter chicken may be unfamiliar to readers. I find recipes for these online, from a search of the desired dish, and you will find some of the online recipes more feasible to prepare than others.

Chapter 14

Exercise and Oxygen

If there was a single treatment that I could give to my cancer patients, one that is free of charge for life, tremendously effective and much safer to have than not have, that would be exercise.

Conversely, I have never seen any more widespread threats to duration and quality of life than these three risky behaviors: reckless driving, recreational substance abuse and a sedentary lifestyle. Reckless driving, fortunately, is relatively rare, as most of us seem to be able to stay in our lane and stop at the red lights, with some remarkable and hair-raising exceptions on our roads and highways.

However, the most common major reckless behavior of our time, sedentary lifestyle, is casually indulged by a majority of 21st century Americans. It is casually indulged, as if there were no victims to this behavior, and as if no harm is expected to come of it. Both assumptions are false, for the following reasons.

The American College of Sports Medicine recommends 150 minutes of exercise per week, broken up into any intervals, of any combination of sports or other movement, _for every living person_. To state the obvious but incomprehensible: This means you -regardless of who you are, your age or your health condition. This recommendation is for Americans of both genders and every last generation even at the extremes, and it is seconded by the Centers for Disease Control.[191] The benefits of long-term exercise have been known throughout human history. Hippocrates warned circa 400 BC, "Eating alone will not keep a man well. He must also take exercise."[192]

I cannot tell you how many sedentary people come in to me amazed when they do not get better, having not comprehended my many exhortations to move and to move frequently, and that their very lives depend on it. Most cancer patients I've met who refused to exercise are now dead.

Yet contemporary Americans are content to leave sports to star athletes and youthful up-and-comers. Only 1 in 5 Americans get the recommended 150 minutes of exercise per week. The rest are literally time bombs for chronic disease. Worse yet, nearly half of high school students – at or near peak physical performance of their lives - do not have a weekly PE class.[193]

The recklessness of not exercising includes a greatly increased risk for Alzheimer's Disease, as exercise is now known as the most effective intervention against onset and progression of Alzheimer's. This poses a threat not only to the wellbeing and quality of life of the individual, but to his safety and that of his family. Likewise, the older woman who chooses not to exercise has increasingly brittle bones, a life-threatening hip fracture waiting to happen. Pre-diabetes and full-blown Type II diabetes are far more prevalent among the sedentary, because lack of exercise impedes blood sugar metabolism.

The most stubbornly sedentary among us may be asking why humans are cursed with exercise as a pre-requisite and co-requisite of good health. I may as well ask why I was cursed with having to nag people to move day after day and decade after decade, in order to help them to get well.

But it is not only these diseases that are very high risk for those with a sedentary lifestyle. Cancer is more likely to strike the sedentary than the non-sedentary. There you have it – the cause of cancer:

In an experiment with mice that were genetically disposed to age prematurely, Mark Tarnopolsky of McMaster University in Ontario divided the mice into two groups. The first group of mice were sedentary. The second group were coaxed on a treadmill three times per week. As expected, the sedentary mice had weaker hearts, thin fur, worse hearing and were shivering in a corner. The healthy mice had sleek coats, ran around their cages, reproduced. However, with regard to cancer, when the mice were sacrificed at the end of the study, half of the sedentary mice had tumors. *None* of the active mice had any tumors at all.[194] None!

There could not be a more stark contrast between a group that's high risk for cancer and a group that's low risk than these sedentary versus active mice.

In my clinic, I exhort people to exercise, and I see all kinds of people. Some are already on their treadmills or other exercise of their choice. The majority tell me they don't exercise much, and that they don't mind going for a walk in the cool weather. Here in the Phoenix area, some consider cool weather to be only the six months from mid-October to early April. So I often hear from patients that they don't want to walk, or haven't been walking because it's too hot.

We look for other forms of exercise that they would be willing to do. We talk about in-home equipment, such as weights and stationary bikes. I tell them that if they live close to a tennis court, they'll play more tennis than me, or if they have a pool, that would be a great option. Very many of my cancer patients find any exercise anathema, and content themselves with making plans for future exercise, rather than getting up today to start moving. Sometimes the late-stage patients decide that they want to spend their days in a wheelchair, rather than the walker that we agreed on. I almost always hate to see this, because, unless they are willing to lift weights and do some aerobic exercises while in the chair, I think the very act of starting to spend time in a wheelchair is going to shorten their lives.

But I am not giving up on any of my patients. The ones in wheelchairs should lift cans of soup or similar weights, for 10 to 20 reps, 3 times per day. The mobile patients should find ways to get to the 150 minutes or more. I exercise about 270 minutes per week, and encourage that for the more fit ones.

Then there are those who insist that, either by laziness or inconvenience or distaste, they will not exercise, I tell them that they need to get into my hyperbaric chamber (HBOT) instead – a more expensive, and possibly not quite as good, alternative to exercise. I recommend this second alternative, the HBOT, so that we can at least accomplish the major benefit that exercise confers in fighting cancer – the benefit of oxygen.

Oxygen uptake is perhaps the best benefit of exercise to a cancer patient. Intense exercise maximizes oxygen uptake. Oxygen at the cellular level is absolutely necessary to nourish our cells, to produce energy, to disassemble and eliminate waste products from our cells, to balance pH and to enhance our immune function. These are essential tasks for the cells of non-cancer and cancer patients alike. These tasks are necessary in the tissue of the cancer patient that we are trying to protect from metastasis, as well as for the tissue already damaged by cancer.

Decreased blood and oxygen flow to vital organs create the setting in which cancer takes its very first stab at the body. In fact, a carcinogen, as defined by Otto Warburg, is a substance that deprives a cell of oxygen, and that causes that cell to convert from aerobic to anaerobic metabolism – the metabolism of cancer cells. This, as biochemist Otto Warburg showed almost 100 years ago, is the initial cause of cancer. He studied many carcinogens, and found that what they had in common, every single one, was the ability to block the cell's uptake of oxygen.

When you consider all the wasted research dollars and time attempting to chase quickly mutating genes to try to associate one more with cancer than others, with vanishing and inconsistent results, the answer was right there all the time, and it is this:

All cancer arises from oxygen deprivation to the cells. All carcinogens have in common that they deprive cells of oxygen. And the first part of the cell damaged is not the DNA, not the genes, not at all. The first part of the cell that is damaged is the mitochondria, site of oxygen utilization and the electron transport chain.

Warburg said, "Cancer has only one prime cause. The prime cause of cancer is the replacement of normal oxygen respiration of body cells by an anaerobic cell respiration.[195]

Cancer seems to be an "obligate anaerobe," that is, that it requires to some extent an oxygen-free environment.[196] To the extent this is true, it makes cancer treatment easier. Our solution: provide oxygen to the patient. How do we do that? If the sedentary patient sits comfortably while hooked up to an oxygen tank, this is not the best way to aerate the body. Only the blood flow and increased lung work induced by exercise will get oxygen efficiently used in the body.

When a normal cell receives increased oxygen, oxidative phosphorylation is the primary metabolic pathway. The electron transport chain is engaged, as well the citric acid cycle, and the mitochondria are able to function in providing energy to the cell, to carry out cell functions, to thrive, eliminate wastes and reproduce.

In a cancerous cell, cellular respiration has converted to anaerobic. When these cells are oxygenated, the remaining normal mitochondria in the previously damaged cell are able to return to normal function and resume metabolism as a normal cell.

Another oxygenating treatment that we do at my clinic is ozone. Whereas oxygen is found in nature as O_2, which is two oxygen molecules covalently bonded together, ozone is O_3. When we combine ozone with the cancer patient's blood, in a short time the O_3 breaks into O_2 and a single O, which then is attracted to and grabs any nearby anaerobes. This includes not only viruses and bacteria, but also cancer cells, destroying them.

Cancer cells have been shown in numerous studies to die in the presence of even a small amount of ozone. One study showed lung, breast and uterine cancers dying at only 0.3 to 0.8 parts ozone per million, with the higher concentration killing more of the cancer cells.[197]

Likewise, hyperbaric oxygen therapy works similarly, yet more effectively. By increasing pressure of room air in a closed environment, more oxygen from the room air is forced into the body and into the blood. By Henry's law, we know that pressure increases the plasma concentration of a gas. In the case of 1.3 atm of room air, the resulting concentration of oxygen in the plasma is increased by 50%.[198] HBOT treatments have been a wonderful boon to natural health care, with very far ranging effects from neurological repair of many kinds, its most lauded and noteworthy effect, to wound-healing and the disruption of cancer metabolism.

Chapter 15

Vitamin C

When I started my medical career, in a conventional osteopathic program, a professor announced to our class to steer very clear of Vitamin C. No reason was given, but a fearful and cautionary tone in the professor's voice made Vitamin C sound like dangerous business! Then earlier this year, at a cancer conference at which I was the only naturopathic physician among mostly medical doctors and a few PhDs, three of the medical doctors spoke fearfully about vitamin C after I gave my talk, in which I had showed results of using it at my clinic for over a decade, and having administered over 30,000 treatments of high-dose intravenous vitamin C. However, to the credit of different MDs present, some took an interest in these results, and were also interested in cooperative and mutually informative discussion on how the breadth of all of medicine, both conventional and natural, could best serve our patients.

That experience was a reminder that there are those in the medical and pharmaceutical professions who fear Vitamin C's powerful ability to compete strongly against the medical cartel's entire arsenal. So let us examine the facts.

Vitamin C is an essential nutrient, meaning that we need it in order to survive and to be well; we cannot rebuild muscle, bone and other tissue without it; we must acquire it from the diet; and we cannot make it in the human body, as most other mammalian species can. Ingestion of vitamin C provides numerous benefits. One of those is the antioxidant function of combatting free radicals, in order to prevent damage to our DNA.

Vitamin C is also essential to the function of our immune systems. It helps also to enable us to absorb iron from food.

The human body is known to require the ingestion of vitamin C in order to produce collagen. We cannot produce collagen without it. The purpose of collagen, as the predominant protein throughout much of the body, is to form the structural basis of and to give strength to our tissue. Bone, cartilage and other tissues are composed of collagen.

Collagen is also necessary to heal wounds. Our skin and GI tract are in nearly constant turnover of tissue. This has to be replaced with the help of Vitamin C to make collagen. The deficiency disease for lack of vitamin C is scurvy. We know of the history of "limey" sailors who took citrus fruit aboard ships to prevent scurvy, a disease that we see more rarely today. Smokers deplete their vitamin C, and we can first diagnosis a pre-scurvy condition in them by easily bleeding gums, gingiva unable to repair in the absence of Vitamin C.

The effect of vitamin C against cancer has been well-documented.

Vitamin C breaks down into hydrogen peroxide among other chemical compounds. Whereas normal cells have catalase, an enzyme that further breaks down hydrogen peroxide into harmless oxygen and water, cancer cells lack that enzyme. In fact, cancer cells are especially interesting because they lack that enzyme. My interest is in the vulnerability that feature confers to cancer cells. Cancer cells are then bathed with hydrogen peroxide after administration of high-dose vitamin C. This seems to stress the cancer cells to the point of cell death.[199]

In 2017 Vitamin C was found effective against cancer stem cells (CSCs). This study showed that Vitamin C was effective in both targeting and sharply reducing the propagation of CSCs.[200]

Several months later, it was found that Vitamin C also accomplished this function of targeting CSCs in the case of certain leukemias, a disease that has been fought primarily with poisons for half a century.[201] [202]

This targeting of cancer stem cells is extremely important, because one of the worst problems in chemotherapy use is the promotion of long-term resistance. In other words, chemotherapy makes cancer stronger in the long run. Cancer stem cells are the cause of this, because they are the residual aspect of cancer not killed by chemotherapy, and are able to generate new and more resilient cancer.[203]

Vitamin C is probably without equal with respect to safety among the most effective natural cancer treatments. If it does have an equal, I would say that it is strenuous daily exercise (Chapter 14).

Ideally, and long sought by conventional medicine, is a "magic bullet," that is, a substance that can distinguish between cancerous and non-cancer cells, in order to target the former, and to leave the latter unharmed.

Vitamin C provides the perfect solution to this problem, for the following reason: A known product of Vitamin C in the extra-cellular fluid, or the fluid that surrounds our cells, is hydrogen peroxide. Now hydrogen peroxide is known to be caustic in its effect on cells. Specifically, it causes oxidative stress, which is damaging to cells, except in this very useful aspect:

Normal cells have an enzyme, catalase, which breaks down hydrogen peroxide to harmless water and oxygen. Cancer cells, however, generally lack this enzyme, and therefore cannot convert hydrogen peroxide to less harmful products. Therefore, the oxidative stress of the hydrogen peroxide seems to overwhelm the cancer cells, and that is what kills them both in vitro (in a petri dish) and in vivo (in a living cancer patient).

But vitamin C is even better than that. An essential nutrient, without which a person would succumb to the life-threatening disease scurvy, vitamin C is necessary for optimal functioning of every bodily system. One specific way in which it is helpful, as discussed above, is this: Vitamin C is necessary to build collagen. I tell my patients that "collagen is the bricks and mortar so to speak that we're made from." Collagen gives our tissues turgor and tensile strength. It is what keeps our gums strong and not weak and bleeding, such as in scurvy. That particular aspect is then useful against one of the several ways that cancer attacks the body. It is useful in preventing the deep invasion of the basement membrane that happens in metastasis. That is, if tissue throughout the body is stronger from plentiful collagen, then it is also less penetrable from metastasizing cancer cells.

And Vitamin C has even more use than that. It is known to strengthen the immune system, and that is something very useful in helping the body to overcome cancer.

Yet Vitamin C has another use. As an essential nutrient to human health, cancer patients who begin to have the vitamin C treatments generally start to feel substantially better within the first couple of weeks. This enables them to begin to exercise or to increase their exercise, which is essential for their overcoming cancer. Exercise oxygenates the body, which has tremendously helpful effects against cancer, as discussed in Chapter 14.

In my clinic, we have found Vitamin C to be most useful as the cornerstone of our natural treatments for cancer. Vitamin C has been shown to kill cancer cells in vivo and in vitro, as we demonstrated in Chapter 7.

However, Vitamin C is *only* a powerful cancer fighter when it is used correctly.

Unfortunately, very unfortunately for many cancer patients, their health insurance will not cover natural treatments for cancer. Even though Vitamin C has a far safer and more effective track record than chemotherapy, the medical cartel has swallowed the insurance industry as well, and the insurance industry has found mutual advantage with the chemo industry in this respect: The more expensive the treatments that insurance companies pay for, the more they can justify charging exorbitant premiums to their customers. Therefore, their profit margin between those two large amounts is also larger (than a scenario with cheap treatments and cheap premiums) and therefore more attractive to insurance companies than a model favoring less expensive medicine.

Vitamin C is far less expensive than chemotherapy. Whereas a single chemotherapy treatment can cost as much as $40,000 or $50,000, a single treatment of Vitamin C costs 1% of that amount or less. If such a practice model as that were to prevail in cancer treatment, insurance companies would not be able to justify charging their customers absurdly high premiums. Then their profit margins would be quite a bit lower.

So even at 1% of the cost of the Cadillac chemotherapy treatments, the insured consumer is often left by their insurance company to pay their entire way with high-dose intravenous Vitamin C (HDIVC) therapy.

Cancer patients who also have to pay enormous deductibles for what is generally inadequate health insurance, are therefore not left in financially robust shape, for the remainder of their battle against cancer that still lies ahead.

So the cancer patient, more often than not, has to pay out of pocket, entirely or mostly for their HDIVC treatments.

This gives rise to a new problem:

Cancer patients often try to save money by spreading out their HDIVC treatments too seldom. And this is a devastating problem:

HDIVC does not work well against cancer if given only seldom. High-dose intravenous vitamin C works better and safer than any known substance against cancer *only* if given regularly, optimally three times per week. Three times per week in my personal experience, and other clinicians before me, is far more effective against cancer than once or twice per week.

Why is this so important? Vitamin C is a water-soluble substance. Unlike Vitamins A, D, E and K, which are fat-soluble vitamins and therefore stay in our body longer, sequestered in the fat, Vitamin C runs through us rather quickly, and needs to be replenished before much time goes on.

Very frequently cancer patients will not appreciate the crucial timing and frequency of vitamin C treatments. So after they start to feel much better, I often hear, "I'll be going on vacation tomorrow, and will see you in a week."

I hate to hear this, because it almost always presages a downturn in their health – a critical window in which cancer can re-establish a strong position during that week away. I will have a much harder time being successful against their cancer after their return. It would be much more prudent of the patient to wait until we have completed 12 weeks of treatment before they take a vacation. I don't even want 4 days between their treatments. Such a period simply gives cancer too much of an opportunity to re-establish itself in the patient's body.

As long ago as Linus Pauling's work with vitamin C and cancer patients, he warned of the problem of trying to use vitamin C seldom in cancer. It must be used frequently, preferably 3 times per week or more. Otherwise, if that is impossible, it would probably be best not to use it at all, and to simply fight cancer with other available means. But that would be a tremendous waste of an opportunity to fight cancer with our one most effective and safest tool. So even when a cancer patient begins to feel substantially better, they should remember that cancer is one of the most difficult and deadly diseases known to man, very thoroughly sequestered and undetectable in the body, and therefore not to interrupt essential treatment with vacations, unless they are absolutely necessary.

Chapter 16

Sodium bicarbonate and alkalinizing strategies

Dr. Tullio Simoncini is a medical doctor in Italy who has done more than anyone to explore the uses of sodium bicarbonate as an alkaline therapy against cancer. It is known that cancer creates and favors an acid environment and because of this, Dr. Simoncini and others have used sodium bicarbonate as an alkaline therapeutic agent against cancer.

The way that acidity seems to protect cancer is not fully understood. One mechanism seems to involve suppression of metastasis. Cancer is known to have acidic extracellular fluid, and that acidity promotes invasion of tumors into the basement membrane, and thereby facilitates metastasis.[204] A study of pH buffers including sodium bicarbonate, showed that acidity was reduced, and that metastasis was inhibited after addition of sodium bicarbonate.[205] [206]

It seems that cytotoxic T-cells, which may attack cancer cells under normal conditions, are inactivated in an acid extracellular fluid.[207] Also, the type of acidity that cancer produces, i.e., lactic acid, stimulates vascular endothelial growth factor (VEGF) and angiogenesis.[208] This can be compared to a highway project, which enables a tumor to build the blood vessels that it needs to bring the nutrients for it to survive. So the tumor creates an environment in which it can then exist comfortably.

At a pH of about 10, sodium bicarbonate is an antidote to this acidity. It can be used clinically in sterile, intravenous form. This is a liquid, sterile baking soda. Sodium bicarbonate ($NaHCO_3$) is well-tolerated, even with frequent repeated dosing. It has been shown that even oral dosing of sodium bicarbonate has raised the pH in the vicinity of tumors and has inhibited tumor growth and metastasis.[209]

As baking soda, we will often recommend that our cancer patients take ¼ to ½ teaspoonful in water orally a few times per day as an adjunct to our therapies. This is not suitable for everybody, and may have repercussions in various organ systems if taken to excess. We are not advising anyone to do this unless they have been a patient at our clinic, and we recommend it to specific individuals. Also, there is risk of aluminum contamination with some available brands of baking soda, so one must be cautious with this.

An important part of our intravenous therapies against cancer is sterile, pure, intravenous baking soda. This is one of numerous anti-cancer nutrients that we use in our intravenous infusions.

Earlier researchers have found a correlation between cancer and candida. In Dr. Simoncini's book, Cancer is a Fungus[210] he notes some similarities between the two. Primarily, both are intractable diseases, each very hard to get rid of. Dr. Simoncini notes that each forms a solid mass of low penetrability, unlike the dispersed forms of bacterial and viral infections in the body or body fluids. Dr. Simoncini notes the problem of surface area in addressing these infections. Whereas bacterial and viral infections are dispersed in the solutions of bodily compartments, and likewise, antibiotics and other anti-microbials dispersed in the same solutions have access to each microbe.

A solid mass on the other hand, is approached by one of two routes: either the most superficial layer of the outer surface, or by way of any blood vessels that course through it.

In the case of a neoplasm, the approach of approximating the most superficial layer has the effect of challenging the survival of the cancer only enough to induce the genetic changes that make the tumor more resilient to further assault by the same or similar agents.

Therefore, a productive route to the core of the cancer, a more threatening assault on its survival, is by way of the bloodstream.

As for whether cancer is fundamentally a kind of fungus, this remains to be determined. However, it is useful to know that not only does sodium bicarbonate disrupt the comfortable environment of tumors, but it also has anti-fungal effect.[211]

For the cancer patient, sodium bicarbonate by intravenous infusion, given by a practitioner who is knowledgeable and experienced in this area, has been helpful to provide an environment that is unwelcoming to cancer. We hope that this will be further researched, so that future clinicians may know optimal dosing and combinations better. Sodium bicarbonate, being one of the most accessible and cost-effective cancer treatments, may become a more commonly accepted practice in cancer therapy.

Chapter 17

Vitamin A

Sometimes I think that our cancer clinic is the only one among our contemporaries that really appreciates the anti-cancer effects of Vitamin A, although Vitamin A has been studied for anti-cancer effect since at least the 1950s.[212] When people come to us after leaving other natural cancer clinics, and if they share a treatment plan with me, Vitamin A is not listed among the supplements recommended by any other clinic that I have seen. Yet hundreds of studies, some of which are cited below, have shown the anti-cancer effects of Vitamin A in its various forms, both *in vitro* (petri dish) and *in vivo* (in the body).

I notice an improved outcome with patients who include Vitamin A in their daily routine over those who forgot that I recommended it. There are many in the latter group, and I don't blame them, because our list of recommended supplements, dietary changes, IV nutrient treatments and lifestyle modifications runs to two or more pages, and must appear daunting to the newcomer.

First let's define Vitamin A. The active metabolite of it, what your body actually uses, is all-trans retinoic acid. But the natural compound of Vitamin A that we use as an oral dietary supplement is retinol. This occurs in nature as retinyl palmitate, which is a retinyl ester. A retinyl ester is retinol linked to a fatty acid. Retinyl palmitate is the most common form of retinol that we see in nature. The form that you get in dietary supplements is most likely retinyl palmitate or possibly retinyl acetate.

This form, retinyl ester in the form of retinyl palmitate, also has shown the greatest effect against cancer cells both in vitro and in vivo. However, all the forms of Vitamin A mentioned here have shown cancer-killing effect, both in the lab and in the body (*in vitro* and *in vivo* in medical parlance), over several dozen studies. Many studies have confirmed anti-cancer effects of all-trans retinoic acid (ATRA). The concentrations have varied from 1 to 30 micromolars. The following are some of the studies that have shown reduced tumor growth in animals after Vitamin A intake. [213] [214] [215] Many human studies have confirmed this, including these studies. [216] [217] [218] [219] [220]

Retinal is most familiar to clinicians who work with Vitamin A. This is the form most important for vision. Severe vitamin A deficiency may lead to immune deficiency and impaired growth in children,[221] and it is most characterized by vision deterioration and finally blindness.[222] [223]

Retinoic acid is of more interest to us because of its effects on immune function and cell differentiation and proliferation. Two forms of this, ATRA and 9-cis-retinoic acid, have been studied for their anti-cancer effects.

When we consume orally retinyl esters, they are converted in the liver to retinol and then to ATRA. Each of those then are transported from the liver to the tissues bound to proteins. When retinyl esters are consumed in the diet, they are taken up with cholesterol and triglycerides and other fatty substances, then packaged into units of transport called chylomicrons. The lymph, which is one third of our body fluid, a one-way circulatory system throughout nearly the entire body, takes those chylomicrons containing vitamin A into the blood. These are then taken to the liver and other tissues. Our LDL cholesterol (mistakenly called "bad cholesterol" by a medical system that doesn't understand its purpose) allows the chylomicrons containing Vitamin A to enter the tissues. There in the tissues of the body, and especially in the liver, the retinyl esters are metabolized to ATRA and retinol. Then in this form they can leave the liver and be carried to tissues that need them by carrier proteins – none of which would be possible without LDL cholesterol.

However, retinyl esters can also be effective against cancer. They are at much higher levels in our blood than other forms of Vitamin A, and can be increased easily by oral administration, unlike the other forms. Retinyl esters are least toxic to the liver, and they occur naturally in foods. However, therapeutic dosing is between 40,000 and 740,000 units per day, for anti-cancer effect, and foods contain a very small fraction of that amount.

Vitamin A is perhaps most helpful against cancer due to differentiation.[224] Colon cancer[225] and some leukemias are some of the cancers that have shown the effect of Vitamin A on differentiation in a beneficial way. [226] [227]

Differentiation can be described this way. Cells of the stomach are specialized (or "differentiated") to be specifically cells of the stomach, or more specifically, parts of the stomach. Cells of the lung are similarly identifiable as lung cells. They can be recognized as such under a microscope. Lung cells, stomach cells, cardiac cells – all different, all identifiable.

Cancer cells on the other hand are not so easily identifiable, because they are not yet differentiated. In more aggressive cancers, pathologists will often note that the cells they see on biopsy are "poorly differentiated." That is, they are not yet specialized into the mature cells of a particular organ. The maturing process or differentiation is a benign process. However, lack of that maturing or differentiation tends to make cancer cells more aggressive; those cells are free to reproduce quickly, to ignore constraints and restraining signals from the rest of the body, and to attain an immortality that becomes a worsening problem for the host organism. In other words, a growing tumor shoves its way against vital organs or against other normal flesh in a way that disregards the needs of the organism or the person, but very much in a way that accommodates its own growth pattern optimally. This is no surprise to us if we consider parasitic behavior from one organism to another. A parasite behaves in its own interest, even though its utter disregard for its host will eventually kill the host and therefore diminish and eliminate the parasite's food supply.

Therefore, the usefulness of Vitamin A as one of the few substances that can induce differentiation makes it a highly valued substance at our clinic. Some of the other easily obtainable natural substances that induce differentiation are Vitamin D, EPA and DHA. Therefore, we often also recommend Vitamin D and cod liver oil or fish oil to our cancer patients, all well-absorbed orally together with Vitamin A, all of those being fat soluble.

The anti-cancer effects of vitamin A have been more extensively studied regarding Vitamin A's inhibition of proliferation.[228] In other words, Vitamin A is good at getting cancer to stop growing: In leukemias,[229] breast cancer,[230] melanoma,[231] prostate cancer,[232] lung cancer,[233] to name several.

Vitamin A has gone through extensive testing on humans, in more than a dozen Phase I and Phase II trials, for a number of cancers, both as a single agent as well as part of multi-nutrient protocols.[234] [235]

Chapter 18

Vitamin D

Let's first define Vitamin D. It is a fat-soluble vitamin, necessary for life and good health. Deficiency in childhood results in a bone-crippling disease known as rickets. In adults, a similar pathology is known as osteomalacia, literally "bad bones." More precisely, the bones are insufficiently mineralized to adequate hardness in these diseases. Vitamin D is essential for stimulation of calcium absorption and for establishing calcium and other minerals in the bones.

Vitamin D3, also called cholecalciferol, is the form of Vitamin D most appreciated for its beneficial effects in the body. It is chemically a hormone. We produce it in the skin on exposure to sunlight. From there it is converted to 25-D3 in the liver, and finally it goes to the kidneys for further action, to produce 1,25-D3, which is the active metabolite. This conversion happens when the body is depleted in the active form, so small amounts are made only on demand by the tissues. Only after it arrives to this active form, 1,25-D3 or 1,25-cholecalciferol, do we finally have a helpful substance.

Like Vitamin A, the active form of Vitamin D is only available as a metabolite, that is, an end-product of the body's processing of food-bound nutrients to a more useful form.

The most promising research on Vitamin D is with the active metabolite, 1,25-D3. This is the form of Vitamin D that has shown greatest effect against cancer.

Many consider this vitamin to be the most important of the natural substances in its effects against cancer. I would not make that claim exactly, but I would prefer not to treat cancer patients without its wonderful help.

1,25-D3 has been shown to be effective against cancer by a number of mechanisms and against a wide range of cancers.

Research has confirmed the essential role that Vitamin D plays in cancer prevention and treatment.[236] [237] [238] [239]

There are randomized, double-blind, placebo-controlled trials showing Vitamin D to be effective against the following cancers:

Melanoma[240]
Cervical cancer[241]
Prostate cancer[242]
Colorectal cancer[243] [244]
Overall cancer risk in women over age 55[245] [246]

As expected, low levels of vitamin D intake had no effect against cancer mortality in this randomized trial.[247]

214

Other smaller studies and animal studies have shown benefit of 1,25-D3 against the following cancers. Here are a few of those:

Gastric cancer[248]
Liver cancer[249]
Breast cancer[250]

Vitamin D metabolites have been shown to have cancer-disrupting effects by several key mechanisms. Vitamin D has been shown to induce differentiation,[251] and apoptosis,[252] to reduce proliferation by effect on signal transduction,[253] to improve intercellular communication by means of gap junction communication preservation,[254] to inhibit angiogenesis,[255] [256] and to inhibit metastasis.[257]

Very promising research abounds regarding synergistic effect between Vitamin D and Vitamin A. Each of these nutrients used alone induces differentiation, which is a way to normalize, cancer cells in a dose-dependent way. The more consumed, the more differentiation observed, in each case. But this differentiation effect was significantly enhanced when Vitamins A and D were combined [258] [259]

It may be even more helpful that the synergistic effect of Vitamin A and D together produced permanently ongoing differentiation of cells, even after both nutrients were discontinued, and even though the differentiation achieved by each of those vitamins used alone was reversible.[260]

This synergy of nutrients should of course be no surprise to those who understand the metabolic pathways in the human body. These pathways illustrate by their meandering routes and intersections that the nutrients are all synergistic in their effects on the cells in our bodies.

It is amazing to me how many people approach our clinic in amazement that we have had better results than other clinics, all without any research grants, hospital affiliations or university affiliations. And a clinic run by a woman no less, when it clearly was supposed to be the case all along that a man would arise from among us to cure cancer. Certainly, I cannot claim to have cured cancer, but we have come a lot further than what was previously done in oncology.

All the amazed people had to do was to look to our longstanding knowledge of biochemistry, and its applied science, nutrition. If you want to achieve the synergy of nutrients in our ongoing fight against the cancer epidemic, you have to make sure that all of the nutrients show up to work in the body. Don't neglect Vitamin A. Don't neglect Vitamin D. Don't neglect Vitamin C. Etcetera. How do you expect a transit system to function if most of the train lines are missing? How do you expect a curtain to continue to hang at your window if most of the threads are not there? This really should not boggle the minds of either clinicians or patients.

Chapter 19

Randomized, placebo-controlled trials of nutrients that kill or prevent cancer

*"The good thing about science
is that it's true
whether or not you believe in it."*

- Astrophysicist Neil deGrasse Tyson

Science is a word used in various contexts much more often than it is defined. Science as an idol is sometimes vehemently defended or just as vehemently derided, without regard for what science actually is. Let's review what constitutes science. Science is the observation of our surroundings, with no or minimal bias, along with the formulation and testing of hypotheses about the nature and function and interactions of our surroundings. That's it; no ideology, no agenda, no strong emotions.

Strictly objective pursuit of science is usually cumbersome, time-consuming and often expensive. As a practical matter, only a researcher or a student has time to pursue small areas of the vastness of all potential science. The rest of us work with what we know of established fact, or assume of established dogma, and most people don't usually take time to re-examine and re-test our cherished hypotheses; we simply act on them.

This haste is prevalent in medicine, because the health insurance industry pressures caregivers to hurry through each patient: physical exams, lab tests or imaging, diagnoses and treatment, all within a short period. Therefore, some leaps of faith are necessary. Doctors just do not have time to test hypotheses with the pressures of the daily workload confronting them. The only expedient way to get through an entire day full of patient appointments is to keep the scrip pad close at hand.

Conventional "standard of care" physicians place their faith in drugs on two things:

(1) the familiar, friendly pharmaceutical representative and the industry behind those drug reps, and

(2) the assumption that at least once in a while the drugs that they sell have been subject to double-blind or at least placebo-controlled trial.

Most cancer patients, and many doctors as well, would be shocked to learn that chemotherapy drugs have not passed the "gold standard" criteria for drug testing: the double-blind, placebo controlled trial. There are two reasons that these double-blind studies are not done for chemotherapy drugs:

(1) With life-threatening illness, it is considered immoral to have a placebo group, in which no treatment is given, and

(2) The one available study that compared a chemotherapy drug to no treatment at all did not appear flattering for the chemotherapy drug or the industry behind it:

That study[261] found that lung cancer patients treated with the chemotherapy drug Docetaxel survived an average of 7.5 months, whereas those receiving merely supportive care with no chemotherapy or other treatment at all survived an average of 4.6 months. If patients knew of this small difference in survival, would they opt to lose their GI tract function, hair, neurological health, cardiovascular health and other wellbeing?

Worse yet, the study found that the group receiving Docetaxel faced the life-threatening conditions of febrile neutropenia and non-hematologic toxicity.[262]

Was all the misery of chemotherapy worthwhile, not to mention the medical bankruptcy that so many families suffer following chemotherapy – was all of that worthwhile, simply in order to gain 3 more months of life?

On the other hand, many nutrients and herbs have been shown effective and safe against cancer.[263] Let's examine some of these cancer treatments that do not damage vitality or quality of life, and some double-blind, placebo controlled trials of those substances.

Gastric and esophageal cancer rates in Linxian, China are among the highest in the world. In 1994, a randomized, placebo-controlled trial was conducted among 29,584 adults, in a general population study.[264] The experimental group was given one of four nutrient treatments for 5.25 years. The doses were the same or double the US recommended daily allowances of the time. It should be kept in mind that the infamous old "RDA" figures were notoriously low, barely enough to prevent vitamin deficiency.

Even with the very low doses of the supplemented nutrients, it was found that the group having Vitamin A and zinc had 62% less gastric (stomach) cancer than the placebo group.

The group receiving beta-carotene (a small component of all of Vitamin A), Vitamin E and selenium had 42% less esophageal cancer than the placebo cohort. These are statistically significant results, and easily adopted interventions that should have been publicized much more broadly around the world, so that the use of Vitamin A, Vitamin E, and mineral use would become more widespread and available.

In another double-blind, placebo-controlled, randomized trial of nutritional supplements,[265] 5141 men were given either a placebo or a single capsule with a very low dose of each of the following sub-optimal forms of generally recognized nutrients:

Vitamin C, alpha-tocopherol (the least effective form of Vitamin E), beta-carotene (one of the least effective forms of Vitamin A), selenium and zinc. They took these daily for 8 years.

There was a statistically significant reduction in the incidence of prostate cancer in the experimental group among the 94% of the men who began the 8 years with a low PSA (<3 micrograms/L). One has to wonder if therapeutic forms and doses of these nutrients had been used, the results may have been even more remarkable.

In another study, which was retrospective, rather than randomized and placebo-controlled, of 37,916 US women, dietary folate and vitamin B-6 .was found to reduce the risk of colorectal cancer over the 10 years of the study.[266]

Vitamin D has been shown to be effective against cancer by a number of mechanisms and against a wide range of cancers. In the previous chapter, we list a number of these studies.

The following randomized, double-blind, placebo-controlled trials show Vitamin D to be effective against the following cancers: cervical cancer,[267] colorectal cancer,[268] [269] melanoma,[270] prostate cancer,[271] overall cancer risk in women over age 55.[272] [273]

A study that found low levels of vitamin D intake had no effect against cancer mortality in this randomized trial[274] may have come to a different conclusion if therapeutic doses had been used.

Other smaller studies and animal studies are mentioned in the previous chapter, which have shown benefit of 1,25-D3, the active form of Vitamin D, against various cancers, such as gastric cancer,[275] liver cancer,[276] and breast cancer.[277]

In the previous chapter, we also examined how Vitamin D and its metabolites have been shown to have cancer-disrupting effects.

Research regarding the synergistic effect between Vitamin D and Vitamin A is looking very promising. Each of these nutrients used alone induces differentiation. Differentiation is essentially a way to normalize the nature and function of cancer cells. It makes stomach cancer cells look and act more like mature, normal stomach cells. Lung cancer cells when differentiated, look more like mature, normal lung cells. The more consumed, the more differentiation observed, for each of the two vitamins. Simultaneous use of Vitamin D and Vitamin A strengthened this effect considerably. [278] [279]

I find it very interesting that the synergistic effect of Vitamin A and D together produced permanently ongoing differentiation of cells, even after both nutrients were discontinued, and even though the differentiation achieved by each of those vitamins used alone was reversible.[280] The strengthening effect of balanced nutrition over lopsided or partial nutrition is a synergy that is not unexpected. A complete nutritional program produces a synergy that is not surprising given the nature and function of the metabolic pathways in the human body.

These metabolic pathways, as filtered by our still limited academic understanding of them, make clear that the nutrients are synergistic in their effects on the cells in our bodies. Just as a well-balanced meal is not all one nutrient alone, optimal nutrition is always multi-faceted.

*   *   *

Double-blind, placebo-controlled trials of any therapy are highly risky in cancer patients due to the higher mortality awaiting the group that fares worse. Clinical trials are ended early if it is clear that one group is benefitting much more than the other cohort, in order for both groups to benefit from the more effective treatment. Therefore, I do not encourage or condone further double-blind, placebo-controlled studies of cancer treatments. The consequences of suffering or death in the less fortunate cohort of cancer patients is unacceptable under any circumstances.

However, now that some of these trials have been done, it is very important that we not allow ourselves to forget the knowledge gained from them, because such knowledge may be decisive in saving the lives of cancer patients.

For optimal dosing of the above nutrients in either cancer treatment or cancer prevention, there is no substitute for consulting a licensed naturopathic physician, in order to evaluate the specific nutritional needs of the individual.

Chapter 20

Randomized, placebo-controlled trials of herbs against cancer

The following studies are some randomized and double-blind, placebo-controlled trials of various botanical medicines against a number of cancers.

Ginger's effect against colorectal cancer

In 2013, a pilot trial of ginger was done with individuals who had been found by genetic markers to be at increased risk of colorectal cancer. The experimental group received supplementation of the common culinary and medicinal herb ginger, the well-known ginger that is available to consumers in markets throughout the world, and that grows easily in the wetter regions of the world.

In the study[281] 20 people were randomized into two groups, those who received 2 grams of ginger or placebo daily, for 28 days. At the end of that time, biopsies were performed of the rectal mucosa. During that time, in the group receiving ginger, biopsies showed that pro-cancerous genes Bax, hTERT and MIB-1 decreased in the crypts of the rectal mucosa. The authors concluded that ginger may decrease proliferation and increase apoptosis and differentiation in colorectal cancer.

Ukrain against colorectal cancer

Ukrain is a derivative of the plant Chelidonium majus, which is the Latin scientific name for the plant greater celandine. It was developed in 1978, and its use was pioneered by Dr. Wassil Nowicky of Ukraine, then Austria. Dr. Nowicky was nominated for the Nobel Prize in Chemistry in 2004 and again in 2006.

A randomized study of 96 colorectal cancer patients found a strong effect of Ukrain against their cancer.[282]

Ukrain against pancreatic cancer

Ukrain showed remarkable effect in the following randomized, controlled trial of pancreatic cancer patients.[283] Of those receiving Ukrain plus low-dose Vitamin C, their rate of remission was remarkable compared to the control group that only received low-dose Vitamin C: 81% survival in the Ukrain group compared to 14% survival in the control group. It would have been interesting if this study had incorporated high dose Vitamin C, as opposed to the 5.4 g Vitamin C that the patients received, which is well below what is generally considered therapeutic dosing. The two year survival was 43% in the Ukrain group, compared to 5% in the control group. At two years of the standard gemcitabine and 5-fluorouracil (Gemzar and 5-FU chemotherapy), 0% survived; all of the chemotherapy patients were deceased. In fact, none of the chemotherapy pancreatic cancer patients survived beyond 19 months. The longest survival in the Ukrain group was 54 months after start of therapy.

Ukrain treatment is well-tolerated, without known side effects.

In fact, in a randomized, controlled study of Ukrain in breast cancer, Ukrain was given along with chemotherapy and mastectomy. The Ukrain patients had better wellbeing and faster recuperation from surgery and better tolerance of their chemotherapy treatments than those who did not.[284]

Other randomized trials of Ukrain in various cancers are described in this meta-analysis.[285]

Combination plant extracts against prostate cancer

A meta-analysis of five randomized trials of various plant extracts, including pomegranate, soy, lycopene, turmeric, green tea and broccoli found the following: Serum PSA levels either stabilized, decreased or rose more slowly in a significant number of men, compared to controls.[286]

One of these studies was a double-blind, placebo-controlled randomized trial involving 199 men with prostate cancer for 6 months. Men in the experimental group were given foods rich in polyphenols, such as pomegranate, green tea, broccoli and turmeric. The experimental group had a 14.7% rise in PSA, as opposed to a 78.5% rise in the placebo group.[287]

Astragalus against lung cancer

226

A meta-analysis of 17 randomized studies, representing 1552 non-small cell lung cancer patients, showed significant improvement in survival for chemotherapy patients having astragalus supplementation over those having chemotherapy alone. This was the case with 1-year, 2-year and 3-year overall survival rates, as well as performance status and tumor overall response rate, as well as tolerance of chemotherapy side effects.[288]

Chapter 21

Hyperthermia

Hyperthermia has become known as a cancer treatment that one must travel to Germany to have. It is assumed that the FDA has prohibited the use of heat as a therapeutic tool. However, if that were the case, then hot baths, hot compresses, saunas, hot tubs, sunbathing, most of Arizona, Palm Springs, CA, heating pads and the like would all have to be confiscated by the FDA. If the time ever comes when the FDA grabs that much power, and even worse, when the American public grants the FDA such power, then it will only be after we are all lobotomized, a day that I do not foresee within the current political culture.

Fortunately, the American public is still permitted to, or rather reserves the right to, apply heat to their own bodies or to have it applied in a clinical setting.

Before considering heat application techniques, let's consider how hyperthermia may be useful against cancer. The National Institutes of Health (NIH) recognizes the use of heat as a therapy that kills cancer cells. In their paper, "Hyperthermia in cancer treatment," the NIH cites studies that show the effect of heat against cancer.[289]

Heat is a promising therapy against cancer, because it exploits an essential difference between normal cells and cancer cells. We always look for such differences, because that realm is where the best anti-cancer therapies are to be found. The temperature difference is this: Cancer cells begin to die at 103 to 104 degrees Fahrenheit, whereas normal cells do not. Cancer cells die at a faster rate between 104 to 111 Fahrenheit.

The mechanism of killing cancer cells is explained by J van der Zee in this way: Cancer cells quickly outgrow their blood supply. So most cancer cells are in an environment of low oxygen and low pH. Those cells seem to be most likely to perish in conditions of high heat.[290] This has been shown to work in cancers of the appendix, bladder, brain, breast, cervix, esophagus, head and neck, liver, lung, melanoma, peritoneum and rectum, as well as sarcomas.

In Phase I, II and III clinical trials, when hyperthermia was combined with radiation therapy, there was an improvement in both tumor reduction as well as duration of life.[291] [292]

Radiofrequency ablation (RFA) is a type of hyperthermia that is used in a targeted way with radio waves to heat and kill cancer cells. Very unfortunately, the FDA has wasted taxpayers' money and killed many cancer patients by harassing some of the few RFA practitioners to the point of having to leave the United States in order to keep practicing. Yet the same United

States government extols RFA through the National Institutes for Health / National Cancer Institute (NIH / NCI).[293] If the taxpayers learned of this, especially those grieving for their lost loved ones, the public fury toward the FDA would likely lead to a sharply decreased role for that agency in its attempted suppression of natural and non-invasive cancer treatments.

Since 1985, the International Journal of Hyperthermia has published peer-reviewed articles on the value of hyperthermia treatments against cancer. This therefore is not brand-new science, and its merits need to be accessible to cancer patients, not suppressed by a corrupted FDA.

The practicalities of using hyperthermia for cancer treatment can range from the quarter-million dollar sophisticated equipment used at the top German cancer clinics, all the way down to an at-home technique of inducing whole body fever, known as constitutional hydrotherapy.

The technique of constitutional hydrotherapy in order to achieve a whole body hyperthermia can, in some individuals, raise the body temperature up to 104 degrees Fahrenheit. Because it may not work so effectively for everyone, I do not recommend this as a stand-alone, at-home treatment for cancer. Rather, a cancer patient should work with a naturopathic physician who is experienced with cancer patients, and who can coordinate hyperthermia into a comprehensive cancer-disrupting program.

Constitutional hydrotherapy is based on the principle of increasing blood flow in order to improve health.

Developed by a naturopathic physician, Dr. O.G. Carroll in the early 1920's, constitutional hydrotherapy became very popular through the 1930's and 1940's and was even adopted by hospitals. Subjective measures of wellbeing as well as objective measures of improved health occur from 2 to 8 hours after constitutional hydrotherapy. White blood cells have been shown to increase in number over that time and last for at least 24 hours. The incidence of colds and flu were found to decrease by 50%.[294]

Instructions for at-home constitutional hydrotherapy may be found at this site: www.MinnesotaNaturalHealth.com/consthydro.htm. Generally, the patient lies comfortably, first face-up, then face-down on a cushioned treatment table. The patient is bundled up in bed sheets and wool blankets, while alternating phases of hot and cold, well-wrung out damp towels are placed over the torso. This in turn creates cycles of vasodilation and vasoconstriction, in order to circulate blood optimally, and to move lymph, in order to help it to carry wastes out the normal elimination routes. Generally, hydrotherapy is done for one hour at a time, but for cancer treatment, we want to achieve a hyperthermia that increases gradually for two hours, is maintained another two hours, and decreases over the following two hours.

However, it is difficult for an individual to prepare their own constitutional hydrotherapy, and it is highly recommended to consult a naturopathic physician or other qualified practitioner, in order to adapt the treatment to the individual and to monitor safety in temperature and total heat and cold exposure.

At our clinic, we generally don't have the personnel availability or the luxury of adequate space to perform a complete 6-hour hyperthermia treatment with constitutional hydrotherapy. There are other options to accomplish this, such as home saunas, in which the body temperature may be raised at the convenience of the individual. The price of home saunas has come down considerably just over the last few years, with some of the portable units selling for $100 to $200 online.

Infrared options are also available for raising body temperature, in the form of heating pads that allow deep penetration of heat, used with adequate protection to prevent burning of the skin. The Biomat and mini-Biomat made by Richway is a brand that has combined infrared heat with safety features, and a number of our patients have used this particular brand, although it must be said that we have no financial relationship with this company other than having purchased and used their equipment since 2014. In all cases, a consult with a licensed naturopathic physician is recommended before using at-home hyperthermia treatments.

Chapter 22

Interview: Opposition to Naturopathic Medicine

<u>Part I: April, 2017</u>

JS: Hi, Dr. Huber.   Thanks for taking time to interview.   I'd like to ask you about opposition to naturopathic medicine.   It seems these days there are two ways to ruin a holiday meal in a big family.   Either discuss left vs. right politics.   Or discuss conventional vs. natural medicine.

CH: So true!   That kind of dispute can heat up quickly.   Opinions are very fixed for a lot of people.

JS: Are you worried about the so-called "Skeptics" and "Science-based medicine" and what they say about natural or naturopathic medicine?   I mean, including you!   You've been attacked too online.   How do you feel about that?

CH: Pharma is understandably worried about its only major competitor: natural medicine and oral supplements sold in health food stores. I mean, look how big Whole Foods is, compared to a decade or two ago. Five decades ago, the whole health food and organic movement just wasn't there at all, except in seedling status. But now it's large and growing fast. So naturally, the FDA, which gets users' fees from their client Pharma, rants about natural supplements. The corruption is so obvious though, they wouldn't dare try to dismantle the supplement industry at this point.

But here's the main reason why I'm not worried. The general public does not need me to tell them which way of living is preferable. Walk into a health food store or a gym, and look around. Then walk into a drug store or a run-of-the-mill supermarket, and look around. Who looks healthier and happier? Which group of people do we all want to look and feel like?

JS: I see what you mean. No contest.

CH: Exactly, no contest. So the so-called skeptics can attack me or attack other individuals. They have really gone after Dr. Oz in a venomous way – and speaking of venomous, there were very strange murders of holistic doctors over the last two years, 2015 mostly.

JS: What was that all about?

CH: At first, it looked like Florida holistic doctors. So I thought maybe it was some pain med disputes. But that turned out to be unlikely. Then it looked like doctors who were critical of vaccines. Then that didn't look right, and it looked like doctors who had taken an interest in GcMAF, which is a Vitamin D-related protein, which some allege to have some effect against cancer. But anyway, if that was the case, and if somebody wanted to eliminate doctors who were working with GcMAF, it backfired, because the murders gave that substance a cachet far beyond what I think it deserves, frankly, and the public took an interest in it, and they're finding it for themselves, for better or worse.

Anyway, where I was going with that was, Pharma can rant till its hoarse – and these keyboard warriors sure do rant! - about natural medicine, supplements, organic food. But at the end of the day, consumers do not want to live a pharmaceutical lifestyle, because it's depressing, fatiguing, painful, humiliating, just all around debilitating. People want to clean up their diet, if only to feel better. They reach for supplements when they know the diet has not been quite as good as it should be. Probably the keyboard warriors sneak them also. And that is exactly what Pharma's big problem is: The American public has not yet been drugged into delirium en masse, probably won't ever be, and still use their minds to question the drug-every-symptom paradigm.

So if naturopathic physicians get attacked over that, we can just shrug and go on. Here's why. The fact is, at least as of 2014, there were NO medical malpractice claims against naturopathic physicians ever in the United States. Ever! Meanwhile, "properly prescribed" drugs kill 128,000 per year. That's more than all the Americans who died in World War I. And that's every year in this country.

So that is the problem for Pharma. They don't have any substantive criticism of us, just angry sniping bloggers. Where is Pharma losing its market share?

To the cemetery more than anywhere. Losing over 100,000 of your loyal customers every year is kind of bad for business, guys. Why not make those drugs less toxic?

There's a website that summarizes these stats: www.bmdiaries.com.

JS: So you don't mind that you've been criticized by the "science-based medicine" crowd.

CH: Well, I have not at all spearheaded the changing zeitgeist the way some others have done. I mean, I report our clinic's results, so the Pharma side is probably thinking: cheeky devil, how dare she. However, none of the accusations I've seen against me are true, and I have a squeaky clean record, no Board complaints, my medical license in good standing the whole decade I've practiced, 5-star ratings from almost all online reviewers. My clinic has an A+ rating with the Better Business Bureau. So that criticism is really not a factor in my work.

Besides, there's nothing science-based about cherry-picking the data one chooses to look at, ignoring all the opposing data, then stooping to angry insults to make arguments. That's the opposite of the scientific method. Intelligent people see past that and realize that those keyboard warriors are just pro-pharma ideologues and hacks. Nothing to worry about in the whole scheme of things.

JS: Thanks, Dr. Huber, mostly for not jumping into the mudslinging pit with them!

CH: That would get ugly! And thank you! I'll get those references to you.

*   *   *

Dr. Huber referred to the following articles in this interview:

http://www.calnd.org/files/CNDA%20Naturopathic%20Doctor%20Safety%20Statistics%20FINAL%202-25-14.pdf
http://ethics.harvard.edu/blog/new-prescription-drugs-major-health-risk-few-offsetting-advantages
https://www.bmdiaries.com/
http://www.healthnutnews.com/about/
http://www.wholefoodsmarket.com/company-info/whole-foods-market-history

Opposition to Natural Medicine

Part 2 of the April 2017 Interview

May 4, 2017

JS: Let's continue our interview from last week. We were talking about the political opposition to natural medicine. I would like to focus more specifically on practitioners such as naturopathic physicians, chiropractors, acupuncturists, and the health food store and supplement industry. What are your thoughts in general about that?

CH: When you consider all those groups together, taken as a whole, we are met with resentment and anxiety from the pharmaceutical industry and the doctors who are most aligned with them – which is most of MDs and DOs. However, there are definitely MDs and DOs who think like we do.

I just want to mention a very notable example: Alan Gaby MD is definitely a leader in alternative / natural medicine in the US. His book Nutritional Medicine is a 1300 page monster, took him 30 years to write, and is a wonderfully useful compendium of data regarding nutritional aspects of disease, symptoms and, on the other hand, good health.

Yet Pharma, and the doctors and hospitals and insurance companies all tied in with Pharma, would rather that none of that information – and none of us – exist, because we are the obstacle to the monopoly that they would have over human health. Actually, the free will of individuals is the ultimate obstacle to full pharmaceutical control of human health.

So I think those are the major actors in the drama. And there is soapboxing and drama in these discussions.

JS: Do you want to talk about that drama, such as when emotions run high between pro-Pharma and anti-Pharma? Or I guess we could say between pro-natural medicine and anti-natural medicine.

CH: I suppose the most virulent word bandied about is "quack," which may be delivered with the implication of duck sounds. However, the word "quack" has an interesting history: It comes from the German "quacksilber" or "quecksilber," originally from Old High German, and means mercury. Well, the interesting aspect of that is that it was the conventional allopathic physicians who trafficked in mercury, not the natural practitioners, because mercury has long been known to be highly toxic – which is not so interesting or useful to those of us in the true healing arts.

Ironically, these days the term "quack" or "quackery" is used dismissively against naturopathic physicians and similar practitioners, with no explanation or particular reason for its use, other than a lazy pejorative that the "skeptic" likes to hurl, similar to other unwarranted expletives.

However, it was the American Medical Association (AMA) and the American Dental Association (ADA) who embraced and defended the use of mercury, even as it fell into wide disfavor among the public even as early as the mid-nineteenth century.

Mats Hanson writes an interesting article about this, in which he points out that then, as now, many conventional doctors used "powerful" treatments in order to try to impress patients, and when they appeared to have symptoms of poisoning, those symptoms could always be blamed on worsening of the original disease.[295]

As someone who works with cancer patients, I can tell you that our era is rife with such antics. Cancer is not nearly so deadly as chemotherapy. Yet when a chemotherapy patient dies, the death certificate lists cancer rather than chemo as the cause of death.

JS: What other points of contention exist between Pharma and natural medicine?

CH: "Science-based medicine" has become a buzzword to indicate synthetic chemicals that are patented. With the patent, these substances can bring a lot of revenue to a company. Now to pass a Phase IV clinical trial, it takes a lot of money changing hands, and Pharma is the only player rich enough to cough up the massive users' fees that are paid to the FDA. The whole arrangement is likely irreparably corrupt. There is little that can be done to change it, because Pharma has over 1500 full-time lobbyists in Congress, which is more than 3 times as many as the number of representatives. That number is also more than the next two biggest industries' lobbyists combined. Now each US representative in Congress faces this problem: It takes massive money to purchase enough advertising to actually win an election; it takes more money than each representative has to spend on a lengthy political campaign. Therefore, they want to and need to take Pharma's money, in order to have a chance of winning. So then the victors, the newly elected, end up voting for legislation that is favorable to Pharma. This of course is frustrating to the public as well as to those of us who practice natural medicine. Because what happens is we in natural medicine tend to get crowded out of legislation, and we find ourselves on the short end of the stick – not adequately reimbursed by health insurance, not reimbursed at all by Medicare.

So then when Pharma talks about "Science-based medicine," what they mean is the medicine that they have paid high prices to run through certain pedigrees. However, they are not referring to medicine that is developed in a scientific way, that is, with careful observation of patient response and reactions.

Herbal medicine is much more based in science, because we have the benefit of studying patient responses over time, enormous time measured in centuries. The herbal monographs let us know in great detail what the observed effects are in patients. This is in contrast to a hastily prepared clinical trial that cuts short careful observation in order to try to rush the latest blockbuster drug to market.

Sometimes this process in Pharma is very sloppy. For example, I was recently waiting in line to board a flight that was delayed. A doctor was speaking nearby on a cell phone, so I heard this half of a conversation:

Hi, this is Dr--------- from -------- Hospital ---------
Research   ....
Oh, hi...............Okay, I need to figure out if Group ----
is on the placebo or on the [medication]...........
So did we get a delivery of the
[medication]?................ Okay, then in that case, I'm
going to assume that group is on the
placebo...............Right............... No, I'm not sure. Did
any of them report any symptoms?........... Yeah, I
wish we could know what they're on. That's the
problem, I just don't know............... Well, that's okay,
I think they must be on the placebo, so just mark them
down as placebo.............. Right, no, I think it'll work
out okay. . . .

I thought, wow, I think we naturopaths must be doing pretty well when our work is compared to that phone dialogue (the half-dialogue that I heard). At least we don't use placebos, unless it seems to be in the patient's best interests. And I would think we would get straight who has which medication!

Closing thoughts:

What are your odds when you have cancer?

Cancer patients who choose naturopathic treatments over chemotherapy are berated by those who had already decided their course of treatment. Naturopathic physicians treat cancer patients, and are berated by oncologists and internet trolls.

Is the war against cancer, or against any alternatives to the status quo?

Cancer patients ask a reasonable question: What are my chances?

A newly diagnosed cancer patient is told: "There is nothing else that works against cancer except chemotherapy and radiation. So you are going to start chemo now." After several chemo drugs are tried, over the course of months to years, the cancer patient must then hear, "There is nothing more that can be done for your cancer." This was after conventional oncology implied to the patient that a cure or at least prolonged remission was possible.

So later, when patients learn the hard way how wrong that is, they get discouraged, distrust these doctors, realize that their cancer is now too strong and too widespread to try anything different, and they go to hospice, and then their death is blamed on cancer, rather than deception and inappropriate treatments.

It just doesn't have to be this way.

We published all the results* of our clinic online from 2009 to 2014, each year, and over the last decade, we still have the best results of any cancer clinic in the world that publishes its detailed results from all consecutively arriving cancer patients. Then when gathering the data each year got to be too detailed and time-consuming, we started surveying patients currently in treatment, and with more focused questions.

Every oncology clinic should publish its results. People need to know their odds. Doctors: Patients have a right to know what you can and cannot do for them. If most of your patients die after a year or two of chemotherapy, then you have the obligation to disclose that to the public, so that people can make informed decisions.

And let them know early enough that they can make the best choices, and get the most effective treatments for their cancer!

---

* www.NatureWorksBest.com
https://natureworksbest.com/wp-content/uploads/2017/01/2016_Cancer_Treatment_Paper.pdf

About the author:

Most doctors who treat cancer don't have much to do with alternative medicine. Most alternative doctors don't see a lot of cancer patients. Colleen Huber, NMD is a Naturopathic Medical Doctor who does both for the last eleven years at her clinic, Nature Works Best Cancer Clinic in Tempe, Arizona. Her clinic has reported their detailed patient results online since 2009.

Dr. Huber was Keynote Speaker at the 2015 Euro Cancer Summit and at the 2016 and 2017 World Congress on Breast Cancer. She is one of the doctors interviewed for the documentary Cancer Can Be Killed on Amazon.

Endnotes

Please note that, although printed links are admittedly cumbersome and tedious to copy, all of the article citations below may be found from a search of key and relevant terms.

Introduction   What choices do cancer patients have?

[1] Euro Cancer Summit. Valencia Spain. 2015 Nov. http://cancer.global-summit.com/europe/2015/scientific-program.php?day=1&sid=1874&date=2015-11-03

[2] Huber C. Defeating cancer requires more than one treatment method. Journal of Cancer Science and Therapy. 2015 Jan. DOI: 10.4172/1948-5956.C1.059. https://www.omicsonline.org/proceedings/defeating-cancer-requires-more-than-one-treatment-method-an-8year-retrospective-case-series-using-multiple-nutritional-and-herbal-agents-2014-update-40692.html

[3] Hyman M. Dangerous spin doctors: 7 steps to protect yourself from deception. http://drhyman.com/blog/2010/10/01/dangerous-spin-doctors-7-steps-to-protect-yourself-from-deception/

[4] Sena M. Fitness industry analysis 2017 – Cost & Trends. www.franchisehelp.com.

[5] Desjardins J. Chart: The largest companies by market cap over 15 years. www.visualcapitalist.com.

Chapter 1   What happens when a person is diagnosed with cancer?

[6] Elizabeth E. https://www.healthnutnews.com/breaking-famous-holistic-naturopathauthor-dies-suddenly/ Aug 2017.

[7] http://www.cnbc.com/2016/06/02/the-worlds-2015-cancer-drug-bill-107-billion-dollars.html

[8] https://www.statnews.com/2016/07/11/for-profit-cancer-centers-advertising/

[9] http://naturopathicstandards.org/naturopathic-medical-education-a-comprehensive-curriculum/

[10] American Association of Physicians and Surgeons. All patients should be guaranteed the following freedoms . . . http://aapsonline.org/patient-bill-rights/

[11] https://www.natonco.org/informed-consent

[12]

http://www.ohchr.org/EN/UDHR/Documents/UDHR_Translations/eng.pdf

Chapter 2   What can you expect when you visit a naturopathic oncologist?

Chapter 3   Why I became a naturopathic physician

[13] Brisson M et al. Exposure to varicella boosts immunity to herpes-zoster: implications for mass vaccination against chickenpox. Vaccine. 2002 Jun 7; 20(19-20). https://www.ncbi.nlm.nih.gov/pubmed/12057605

[14] Hyman M. Dangerous spin doctors: 7 steps to protect yourself from deception. www.drhyman.com.

[15] Light D. New prescription drugs: a major health risk with few offsetting advantages. Harvard University Center for Ethics. Jun 2014. https://ethics.harvard.edu/blog/new-prescription-drugs-major-health-risk-few-offsetting-advantages

[16] Crigger M et al. How many Americans have died in US wars? PBS News Hour. May 2015. http://www.pbs.org/newshour/updates/many-americans-died-u-s-wars/

[17] www.ismp.org/quarterwatch.

[18] Huber C, Waters R. Cholesterol and diet in cancer survivors: a double-blind, retrospective case series of 255 patients in a naturopathic clinic. Cancer Science: Open Access. Jun 2015.
http://scientonline.org/fulltext/cholesterol-and-diet-in-cancer-survivors-a-double-blind-retrospective-case-series-of-255-cancer-patients-in-a-naturopathic-clinic/21185

[19] Jaxen J. Kennedy Jr. exposes corporate media as Youtube cuts off independent voices. Apr 2017.
http://www.jeffereyjaxen.com/blog/kennedy-jr-exposes-corporate-media-as-youtube-cuts-off-independent-voices

[20] Baker S. Americans are increasingly using complementary and alternative medicine. NaturalNews.com. Oct.2009.
http://www.naturalnews.com/027291_americans_health_survey.html

[21] National Institutes of Health. National center for Complementary and Integrative Health. The use of complementary and alternative medicine in the United States.
https://nccih.nih.gov/research/statistics/2007/camsurvey_fs1.htm.

Chapter 4   Cancer politics: A cynical view of the current state of cancer treatment in the US

Chapter 5   Frequently asked questions

Chapter 6   Risks and benefits of chemotherapy vs. natural treatments

[22] Blumen H, Fitch K. et al. Comparison of treatment costs for breast cancer, by tumor stage and type of service. American Health Drug Benefits. 2016 Feb; 9(1):23-32.
https://www.ncbi.nlm.nih.gov/pmc/articles/PMC4822976/

[23] StudentDoctor.net. Pathology movie coming to theaters.
https://forums.studentdoctor.net/threads/pathology-movie-coming-to-theatres.1158889/ Aug 2015.

[24] Spruill L. Pathologic assessment of breast core biopsies: limitations and pitfalls. 6th World Congress on Breast Cancer and Therapy. October 16 - 18, 2017. San Francisco, USA. https://breastcancer.conferenceseries.com/america/scientific-program#tab1

[25] https://nd.az.gov/

[26] Huber C. Defeating cancer requires more than one treatment method. 2016 Dec. https://natureworksbest.com/wp-content/uploads/2017/01/2016_Cancer_Treatment_Paper.pdf

[27] Morgan G et al. The contribution of cytotoxic chemotherapy to 5-year survival in adult malignancies. Clin Oncol 2004 Dec. 16(8). 549-60. https://www.ncbi.nlm.nih.gov/pubmed/15630849

[28] Karagiannis G, Pastoriza J, et al. Neoadjuvant chemotherapy induces breast cancer metastasis through a TMEM-mediated mechanism. Science Translational Medicine. 05 Jul 2017. Vol 9, Issue 397. https://www.ncbi.nlm.nih.gov/pmc/articles/PMC5592784/

[29] Huber C Defeating cancer requires more than one treatment methods: a 10-year retrospective case series using multiple nutritional and herbal agents, 2016 update. www.NatureWorksBest.com

[30] Naturopathic Cancer Society. Naturopathic Medicine works best to eliminate bladder cancer, breast cancer, colorectal cancer, etc. www.NatOnco.org.

Chapter 7   Defeating cancer requires more than one treatment method

[31] Boik, John. Natural Compounds in Cancer Therapy. Oregon Medical Press. 2001; p.2.

[32] Huber, Colleen. Naturopathic Medical Education: Does it Measure Up? A curriculum comparison among three naturopathic medical colleges, Yale University School of Medicine and Arizona College of Osteopathic Medicine, conducted at Southwest College of Naturopathic Medicine, April 14, 2005.

[33] Huber C. Naturopathic Medical Education: A Comprehensive Curriculum. NaturopathicStandards.org. 2015. http://naturopathicstandards.org/naturopathic-medical-education-a-comprehensive-curriculum/

[34] Warburg, O. The Metabolism of Tumors [book] 1926. https://www.ncbi.nlm.nih.gov/pmc/articles/PMC2140820/pdf/519.pdf

[35] Chan J, Wang F, Holly E. Sweets, sweetened beverages, and risk of pancreatic cancer in a large population based case-control study. Cancer Causes & Control. 2009 Aug; 20(6): 835-46. https://www.ncbi.nlm.nih.gov/pmc/articles/PMC2694313/

[36] Rossi M, Lipworth L, et al. Dietary glycemic index and glycemic load and risk of pancreatic cancer: a case-control study. Ann Epidemiol. 2010 Jun. 20(6): 460-465. https://www.ncbi.nlm.nih.gov/pubmed/20470973

[37] Mueller N, Odegaard A, et al. Soft drink and juice consumption and risk of pancreatic cancer: the Singapore Chinese Health Study. Cancer Epidemiol Biomarkers Prev. 2010 Feb. 19(2). 447-455. https://www.ncbi.nlm.nih.gov/pubmed/20142243

[38] Larsson S, Berqkvist L, et al. Consumption of sugar and sugar-sweetened foods and the risk of pancreatic cancer in a prospective study. Am J Clin Nutr. 2006 Nov. 84(5). 1171-1176. https://www.ncbi.nlm.nih.gov/pubmed/17093171

[39] Tavani A, Giordano L, et al. Consumption of sweet foods and breast cancer risk in Italy. Ann Oncol. 2006 Feb. 17(2). 341-345. https://www.ncbi.nlm.nih.gov/pubmed/16249211

[40] Larsson, S, Bergkvist L, Wolk A. Glycemic load, glycemic index and breast cancer risk in a prospective cohort of Swedish women. Int J Cancer. 2009 Jul 1; 125(1): 153-7. https://www.ncbi.nlm.nih.gov/pubmed/19319984

[41] Wu A, Yu M, Tseng C. et al. Dietary patterns and breast cancer risk in Asian American women. Am J Clin Nutr. 2009 Apr; 89(4): 1145-54. https://www.ncbi.nlm.nih.gov/pubmed/19211822

[42] Bradshaw P et al. Consumption of sweet foods and breast cancer risk: a case-control study of women on Long Island, New York.

Cancer Causes Control. 2009 Oct. 20(8). 1509-1515.
https://www.ncbi.nlm.nih.gov/pmc/articles/PMC4109805/

[43] Freedland S, Aronson, W. Dietary intervention strategies to modulate prostate cancer risk and prognosis. Curr Opin Urol. 2009 May; 19(3): 263-7. https://www.ncbi.nlm.nih.gov/pubmed/19300265

[44] Drake I, Sonestedt E, et al. Dietary intakes of carbohydrates in relation to prostate cancer risk: a prospective study in the Malmo Diet and Cancer cohort. Am J Clin Nutr. 2013 Dec. 96(6): 1409-18. https://www.ncbi.nlm.nih.gov/pubmed/23134882

[45] Ikeda F, Doi Y, et al. Hyperglycemia increases risk of gastric cancer posed by Helicobacter pylori infection: a population-based cohort study. Gastroenterology. 2009 Aprei(4): 1234-41. https://www.ncbi.nlm.nih.gov/pubmed/19236964

[46] Bertuccio P, Praud D, et al. Dietary glycemic load and gastric cancer risk in Italy. Br J Cancer. 2009 Feb 10; 100(3): 558-61. https://www.ncbi.nlm.nih.gov/pubmed/19190635

[47] Wang B, Bobe G, et al. High sucrose diets promote intestinal epithelial cell proliferation and tumorigenesis in APC mice by increasing insulin and IGF-1 levels. Nutr Cancer. 2009; 61(1): 81-93. https://www.ncbi.nlm.nih.gov/pubmed/19116878

[48] Wang B, Bobe G, et al. Dietary carbohydrate source alters gene expression profile of intestinal epithelium in mice. Nutr Cancer. 2009; 61(1): 146-55. https://www.ncbi.nlm.nih.gov/pubmed/19116885

[49] Nayak S, Sasi M, et al. A case control study of roles of diet in colorectal carcinoma in a South Indian population. Asian Pac J Cancer Prev. 2009 Oct-Dec. 10(4). 565-568. https://www.ncbi.nlm.nih.gov/pubmed/19827870

[50] Williams C, Satia J, et al. Dietary patterns, food groups, and rectal cancer risk in whites and African-Americans. Cancer Epidemiol Biomarkers Prev. 2009 May. 18(5). 1552-1561. https://www.ncbi.nlm.nih.gov/pubmed/19423533

[51] Augustin L, Polesel J, et al. Dietary glycemic index, glycemic load and ovarian cancer risk: a case-control study in Italy. Ann Oncol.

2003 Jan; 14(1): 78-84.
https://www.ncbi.nlm.nih.gov/pubmed/12488297

[52] Silvera S, Jain M, et al. Glycaemic index, glycaemic load and ovarian cancer risk: a prospective cohort study. Public Health Nutr. 2007 Octo. 10(10). 1076-1081.
https://www.ncbi.nlm.nih.gov/pubmed/17381931

[53] King M, Chandran U, et al. Consumption of sugary foods and drinks and risk of endometrial cancer. Cancer Causes Control. 2013 Jul 24(7) 1427-1436. https://www.ncbi.nlm.nih.gov/pmc/articles/PMC3683350/

[54] Mulholland H, Murray L, et al. Dietary glycaemic index, glycaemic load and endometrial and ovarian cancer risk: a systematic review and meta-analysis. Br J Cancer. 2008 Aug 5. 99(3). 434-441.
https://www.ncbi.nlm.nih.gov/pmc/articles/PMC2527795/

[55] Fedirko V, Lukanova A, et al. Glycemic index, glycemic load, dietary carbohydrate, and dietary fiber intake and risk of liver and biliary tract cancer in Western Europeans. Ann Oncol. 2013 Feb. 24(2). 543-553. https://www.ncbi.nlm.nih.gov/pubmed/23123507

[56] Moerman C, Bueno de Mesquita H, et al. Consumption of foods and micronutrients and the risk of cancer of the biliary tract. Prev Med. 1995 Nov. 24(6). 591-602.
https://www.ncbi.nlm.nih.gov/pubmed/8610083

[57] Creagan E, Moertel C, et al. Failure of high-dose Vitamin C (ascorbic acid) therapy to benefit patients with advanced cancer. A controlled trial. New Engl J Med 1979 Sep 27. 301(13): 687-90.
https://www.ncbi.nlm.nih.gov/pubmed/384241

[58] Moertel C, Fleming T, et al. High-dose vitamin C versus placebo in the treatment of patients with advanced cancer who have had no prior chemotherapy. A randomized double-blind comparison. New Engl J Med. 1985 Jan 17; 312(3): 137-41.
https://www.ncbi.nlm.nih.gov/pubmed/3880867

[59] Cameron E, Campbell A. The Orthomolecular treatment of cancer: II. Clinical trial of high-dose ascorbic acid supplements in advanced human cancer. Chem Biol Interact. 1974; 9: 285-315.
http://www.cellmedsoc.org/research_archive/NHC/studien_pdf/old/the_orthomolecular_treatment_of_cancer.pdf

[60] Cameron E, Pauling L. Supplemental ascorbate in the supportive treatment of cancer: prolongation of survival times in terminal human cancer. Proc Natl Acad Sci. 1976. 73. 3685-89. https://www.ncbi.nlm.nih.gov/pubmed/1068480

[61] Cameron E., Pauling L. Supplemental ascorbate in the supportive treatment of cancer: re-evaluation of prolongation of survival times in advanced human cancer. Proc Natl Acad Sci. 1978 Sep; 75(9): 4538-42.
[62] Bram S, Froussard P, Guichard M, et al. Vitamin C preferential toxicity for malignant melanoma cells. Nature 1980 Apr 17; 284(57):629-31. https://www.ncbi.nlm.nih.gov/pubmed/279931

[63] Leung P, Miyashita K, et al. Cytotoxic effect of ascorbate and its derivatives on cultured malignant and non-malignant cell lines. Anticancer Res. 1993 Mar-Apr; 13(2): 475-80. https://www.ncbi.nlm.nih.gov/pubmed/8517665

[64] Sakagami H, Satoh K, et al. Apoptosis-inducing activity of vitamin C and vitamin K. Cell Mol. Biol 2000 Feb; 46(1): 129-43. https://www.ncbi.nlm.nih.gov/pubmed/10726979

[65] Chen Q, Espey M, et al. Pharmacologic ascorbic acid concentrations selectively kill cancer cells: action as a pro-drug to deliver hydrogen peroxide to tissues. Proc Natl Acad Sci. 2005 Sep; 102(38): 13604-09. https://www.ncbi.nlm.nih.gov/pubmed/16157892

[66] Padayatty S., Sun H, et al. Vitamin C pharmacokinetics: implications for oral and intravenous use. Ann Intern Med 2004 Apr 6;140(7): 533-37. https://www.ncbi.nlm.nih.gov/pubmed/15068981

[67] Chen Q, Espey M, Krishna M, et al. Pharmacologic ascorbic acid concentrations selectively kill cancer cells: action as a pro-drug to deliver hydrogen peroxide to tissues. Proc Natl Acad Sci. 2005 Sep. 102(38): 13604-09. https://www.ncbi.nlm.nih.gov/pubmed/16157892

[68] Padayatty S, Riordan H, et al. Intravenously administered vitamin C as cancer therapy: three cases. Canadian Med Assn J. 2006 Mar 28; 174(7): 937-42. https://www.ncbi.nlm.nih.gov/pmc/articles/PMC1405876/

253

[69] Akiyama M, Nakamura M. Bone regeneration and neovascularization processes in a pellet culture system for periosteal cells. Cell Transplant. 2009 Apr 15.
https://www.ncbi.nlm.nih.gov/pubmed/19622231

[70] Yogeeta S, Gnanapragasam A, et al. Synergistic salubrious effect of ferulic acid and ascorbic acid on membrane-bound phosphatases and lysosomal hydrolases during experimental myocardial infarction in rats. Life Sci. 2006 Dec.23; 80(3): 258-63.
https://www.ncbi.nlm.nih.gov/pubmed/17045618

[71] Lin Y, Tan F, et al. Synthesis and characterization of collagen/hyaluronan/chitosan composite sponges for potential biomedical applications. Acta Biomater. 2009 Apr 2.
https://www.ncbi.nlm.nih.gov/pubmed/19427824

[72] Petrella B. Assessment of local proteolytic milieu as a factor in tumor invasiveness and metastasis formation: in vitro collagen degradation and invasion assays. Methods Mol Biol 2009; 511:75-84.
https://www.ncbi.nlm.nih.gov/pubmed/19347293

[73] Penna-Martinez M, Ramos-Lopez E., et al. Vitamin D receptor polymorphisms in differentiated thyroid carcinoma. Thyroid. 2009 Jun; 19(6): 623-8. https://www.ncbi.nlm.nih.gov/pubmed/19499989

[74] Robien K, Cutler G, et al. Vitamin D intake and breast cancer risk in post-menopausal women: the Iowa Women's Health Study. Cancer Causes Control. 2007 Sep; 18(7): 775-82.
https://www.ncbi.nlm.nih.gov/pubmed/17549593

[75] Epstein E, Lindqvist P, et al. A population-based cohort study on sun habits and endometrial cancer. Br J Cancer. 2009 Jun 23.
https://www.ncbi.nlm.nih.gov/pmc/articles/PMC2720243/

[76] Giovannucci E. The epidemiology of vitamin D and cancer incidence and mortality: a review. Cancer Causes Control. 2005 Mar; 16(2): 83-95. https://www.ncbi.nlm.nih.gov/pubmed/15868450

[77] Wei M, Garland C, et al. Vitamin D and prevention of colorectal adenoma: a meta-analysis. Cancer Epidemiol Biomarkers Prev. 2008 Nov; 17(11): 2958-69.
https://www.ncbi.nlm.nih.gov/pubmed/18990737

[78] Garland C, Gorham E, et al. Vitamin D for cancer prevention: global perspective. Ann Epidem 2009 Jul;19(7):468-83. https://www.ncbi.nlm.nih.gov/pubmed/19523595

[79] Giovannucci E. Vitamin D and cancer incidence in the Harvard cohorts. Ann Epidem. 2009 Feb 19(2): 84-8. https://www.ncbi.nlm.nih.gov/pubmed/18291673

[80] Shen M, Yen A. Nicotinamide cooperates with retinoic acid and 1,25 dihydroxyvitamin D(3) to regulate cell differentiation and cell cycle arrest of human myeloblastic leukemia cells. Oncology 2009; 76(2): 91-100. https://www.ncbi.nlm.nih.gov/pubmed/19127080

[81] Kizildag S, Ates H. Treatment of K562 cells with 1,25 dihydroxyvitamin D(3) induces distinct alterations in the expression of apoptosis-related genes BCL-2, BAX, BCL(XL) and p21. Ann Hematol. 2009 May 28. https://www.ncbi.nlm.nih.gov/pubmed/19475409

[82] Wu W, Zhang X, et al. 1alpha, 25 dihydroxyvitamin D(3) anti-proliferative actions involving vitamin D receptor-mediated activation of MAPK pathways and AP-1/p21 (wafl) upregulation in human osteosarcoma. Cancer Lett. 2007 Aug 28. 254(1): 75-86. https://www.ncbi.nlm.nih.gov/pubmed/17412493

[83] Fujioka T, Suzuki Y, et al. Prevention of renal cell carcinoma by active vitamin D(3). World J Surg. 2000 Oct; 24(10): 1205-10. https://www.ncbi.nlm.nih.gov/pubmed/11071463

[84] Bao B, Yao J, et al. 1alpha, 25-dihydroxyvitamin D3 suppresses interleukin-8-mediated prostate cancer cell angiogenesis. Carcinogenesis. 2006 Sep; 27(9): 1883-93. https://www.ncbi.nlm.nih.gov/pubmed/16624828

[85] Chung I, Han G, et al. Role of Vitamin D receptor in the antiproliferative effects of calcitriol in tumor-derived endothelial cells and tumor angiogenesis in vivo. Cancer Res. 2009 Feb 1; 69(3):. 967-75. https://www.ncbi.nlm.nih.gov/pubmed/19141646

[86] Yudoh K, Matsuno H, et al. 1alpha, 25-dihydroxyvitamin D3 inhibits in vitro invasiveness through the extracellular matrix and in vivo pulmonary metastasis of mouse melanoma. J Lab Clin Med.

1999 Feb 133(2): 120-8.
https://www.ncbi.nlm.nih.gov/pubmed/9989763

[87] Mora J, Iwata M, et al. Vitamin effects on the immune system: vitamins A and D take centre stage. Nat Rev Immunol. 2008 Sep; 8(9): 685-98. https://www.ncbi.nlm.nih.gov/pubmed/19172691

[88] Guan J, Zhang H, et al.. Retinoic acid inhibits pancreatic cancer cell migration and EMT through the down-regulation of IL-6 in cancer associated fibroblast cells.
Cancer Lett. 2013 Dec 11.
https://www.ncbi.nlm.nih.gov/pubmed/24334138

[89] Montrone M, Martorelli D, et al. Retionoids as critical modulators of immune functions: new therapeutic perspectives for old compounds. Endocr Metab Immune Disorder Drug Targets. 2009 June; 9(2): 133-31. https://www.ncbi.nlm.nih.gov/pubmed/19519462

[90] Kusmartzev S, Su Z, et al. Reversal of myeloid cell-mediated immunosuppression in patients with metastatic renal cell carcinoma. Clin Cancer Res.2008 Dec 15; 14(24): 8270-8.
https://www.ncbi.nlm.nih.gov/pubmed/19088044

[91] Okuno M, Kojima S, et al. Retinoids in cancer chemoprevention. Curr Cancer Drug Targets. 2004 May; 4(3): 285-98.
https://www.ncbi.nlm.nih.gov/pubmed/11574627

[92] Wu Q, Dawon, M, et al. Inhibition of trans-retinoic acid-resistant human breast cancer cell growth by retinoid X receptor-selective retinoids. Mol Cell Biol 1997 Nov; 17(11): 6598-608.
https://www.ncbi.nlm.nih.gov/pubmed/9343423

[93] Cannell J, Vieth R, et al. Cod liver oil, vitamin A toxicity, frequent respiratory infections and the vitamin D deficiency epidemic. Ann Otol, Rhinol, Laryngol. 2008 Nov; 117(11): 864-70.
http://journals.sagepub.com/doi/abs/10.1177/000348940811701112

[94] Makishima M, Honma Y, et al. Effects of inhibitors of protein tyrosine kinase activity and/or phosphatidylinositol turnover on differentiation of some leukemia myelomonocytic leukemia cells. Leukemia Res 1991; 15(8): 701-08.
http://www.lrjournal.com/article/0145-2126(91)90072-2/pdf

[95] Sokolski J, Sartorelli A. Induction of the differentiation of HL-60 promyelocytic leukemia cells by nonsteroidal anti-inflammatory agents in combination with low levels of vitamin D3. Leuk Res 1998 Feb; 22(2): 153-61. https://www.ncbi.nlm.nih.gov/pubmed/9593472

[96] Shen M, Yen A. Nicotinamide cooperates with retinoic acid and 1,25 dihydroxyvitamin D(3) to regulate cell differentiation and cell cycle arrest of human myeloblastic leukemia cells. Oncology 2009; 76(2): 91-100. https://www.ncbi.nlm.nih.gov/pubmed/19127080

[97] Kulp K, Montgomery J, et al. Essiac and Flor-essence herbal tonics stimulate the in vitro growth of human breast cancer cells. Breast Cancer Res Treat. 2006 Aug; 98(3). 249-59. https://link.springer.com/article/10.1007/s10549-005-9156-x

[98] Seely D, Kennedy D, et al. In vitro analysis of the herbal compound Essiac. Anticancer Res. 2007 Nov-Dec; 27(6B). 3875-82. https://www.ncbi.nlm.nih.gov/pubmed/18225545

[99] Leonard S, Keil D, et al. Essiac tea: scavenging of reactive oxygen species and effects on DNA damage. J Ethnopharmacol. 2006 Jan 16; 103(2): 288-96. https://www.ncbi.nlm.nih.gov/pubmed/16226859

[100] Ottenweller J, Putt K, et al. Inhibition of prostate cancer cell proliferation by Essiac. J Altern Complement Med. 2004 Aug; 10(4): 687-91. https://www.ncbi.nlm.nih.gov/pubmed/15353028

[101] Proefrock K. Botanical considerations for lung cancer patients. (Lecture) Southwest Conference on Botanical Medicine. Tempe, AZ USA. 2001. https://www.botanical-medicine.org/Botanical-Medicine-Conferences/2001-Southwest-Conference-on-Botanical-Medicine/Botanical-Considerations-for-Lung-Cancer

[102] Huber C. Optimal Diets for Cancer Patients: 8 years of cancer survivors' best choices. NatureWorksBest.com. Dec.2015. https://natureworksbest.com/wp-content/uploads/2015/12/Optimal-Diets-for-Cancer-Patients.pdf

[103] Huber C. Extroversion, expression and appreciation among cancer patients. NatureWorksBest.com.

[104] Huber C. Defeating cancer requires more than one treatment method. https://natureworksbest.com/wp-content/uploads/2017/01/2016_Cancer_Treatment_Paper.pdf
[105] Ibid. Huber. Optimal Diets for Cancer Patients. https://natureworksbest.com/wp-content/uploads/2015/12/Optimal-Diets-for-Cancer-Patients.pdf

[106] Ibid. Huber. Extroversion, expression and appreciation among cancer patients. NatureWorksBest.com

[107] Jones, M, Young, R, Scully R. Endometrial adenocarcinoma with a component of giant cell carcinoma. Int J Gynecol Pathol. 1991; 10(3): 260-270. https://www.ncbi.nlm.nih.gov/pubmed/1917275

Chapter 8   Glycemic restriction in cancer patients

[108] Chan J, Wang F, Holly E. Sweets, sweetened beverages, and risk of pancreatic cancer in a large population based case-control study. Cancer Causes & Control. 2009 Aug; 20(6): 835-46. https://www.ncbi.nlm.nih.gov/pmc/articles/PMC2694313/

[109] Rossi M et al. Dietary glycemic index and glycemic load and risk of pancreatic cancer: a case-control study. Ann Epidemiol. 2010 Jun. 20(6): 460-465. https://www.ncbi.nlm.nih.gov/pubmed/20470973

[110] Mueller N, Odegaard A, et al. Soft drink and juice consumption and risk of pancreatic cancer: the Singapore Chinese Health Study. Cancer Epidemiol Biomarkers Prev. 2010 Feb. 19(2). 447-455. https://www.ncbi.nlm.nih.gov/pubmed/20142243

[111] Larsson S. Berqkvist L, et al. Consumption of sugar and sugar-sweetened foods and the risk of pancreatic cancer in a prospective study. Am J Clin Nutr. 2006 Nov. 84(5). 1171-1176. https://www.ncbi.nlm.nih.gov/pubmed/17093171

[112] Tavani A, Giordano L, et al. Consumption of sweet foods and breast cancer risk in Italy. Ann Oncol. 2006 Feb. 17(2). 341-345. https://www.ncbi.nlm.nih.gov/pubmed/16249211
[113] Larsson, S, Bergkvist L, et al. Glycemic load, glycemic index and breast cancer risk in a prospective cohort of Swedish women. Int J

Cancer. 2009 Jul 1; 125(1): 153-7.
https://www.ncbi.nlm.nih.gov/pubmed/19319984

[114] Wu A, Yu M, et al. Dietary patterns and breast cancer risk in Asian American women. Am J Clin Nutr. 2009 Apr; 89(4): 1145-54.
https://www.ncbi.nlm.nih.gov/pubmed/19211822

[115] Bradshaw P et al. Consumption of sweet foods and breast cancer risk: a case-control study of women on Long Island, New York. Cancer Causes Control. 2009 Oct. 20(8). 1509-1515.
https://www.ncbi.nlm.nih.gov/pmc/articles/PMC4109805/

[116] Freedland S, Aronson, W. Dietary intervention strategies to modulate prostate cancer risk and prognosis. Curr Opin Urol. 2009 May; 19(3): 263-7. https://www.ncbi.nlm.nih.gov/pubmed/19300265

[117] Drake I, Sonestedt E, et al. Dietary intakes of carbohydrates in relation to prostate cancer risk: a prospective study in the Malmo Diet and Cancer cohort. Am J Clin Nutr. 2013 Dec. 96(6): 1409-18.
https://www.ncbi.nlm.nih.gov/pubmed/23134882

[118] Ikeda F, Doi Y, et al. Hyperglycemia increases risk of gastric cancer posed by Helicobacter pylori infection: a population-based cohort study. Gastroenterology. 2009 Aprei(4): 1234-41.
https://www.ncbi.nlm.nih.gov/pubmed/19236964

[119] Bertuccio P, Praud D, et al. Dietary glycemic load and gastric cancer risk in Italy. Br J Cancer. 2009 Feb 10; 100(3): 558-61.
https://www.ncbi.nlm.nih.gov/pubmed/19190635

[120] Wang B, Bobe G, et al. High sucrose diets promote intestinal epithelial cell proliferation and tumorigenesis in APC mice by increasing insulin and IGF-1 levels. Nutr Cancer. 2009; 61(1): 81-93.
https://www.ncbi.nlm.nih.gov/pubmed/19116878

[121] Wang B, Bobe G, et al. Dietary carbohydrate source alters gene expression profile of intestinal epithelium in mice. Nutr Cancer. 2009; 61(1): 146-55. https://www.ncbi.nlm.nih.gov/pubmed/19116885

[122] Nayak S, Sasi M, et al. A case control study of roles of diet in colorectal carcinoma in a South Indian population. Asian Pac J Cancer Prev. 2009 Oct-Dec. 10(4). 565-568.
https://www.ncbi.nlm.nih.gov/pubmed/19827870

[123] Williams C, Satia J, et al. Dietary patterns, food groups, and rectal cancer risk in whites and African-Americans. Cancer Epidemiol Biomarkers Prev. 2009 May. 18(5). 1552-1561.
https://www.ncbi.nlm.nih.gov/pubmed/19423533

[124] Augustin L, Polesel J, et al. Dietary glycemic index, glycemic loan and ovarian cancer risk: a case-control study in Italy. Ann Oncol. 2003 Jan; 14(1): 78-84.
https://www.ncbi.nlm.nih.gov/pubmed/12488297

[125] Silvera S, Jain M, et al. Glycaemic index, glycaemic load and ovarian cancer risk: a prospective cohort study. Public Health Nutr. 2007 Octo. 10(10). 1076-1081.
https://www.ncbi.nlm.nih.gov/pubmed/17381931

[126] King M, Chandran U, et al. Consumption of sugary foods and drinks and risk of endometrial cancer. Cancer Causes Control. 2013 Jul 24(7) 1427-1436.
https://www.ncbi.nlm.nih.gov/pmc/articles/PMC3683350/

[127] Mulholland H, Murray L, et al. Dietary glycaemic index, glycaemic load and endometrial and ovarian cancer risk: a systematic review and meta-analysis. Br J Cancer. 2008 Aug 5. 99(3). 434-441.
https://www.ncbi.nlm.nih.gov/pmc/articles/PMC2527795/

[128] Fedirko V, Lukanova A, et al. Glycemic index, glycemic load, dietary carbohydrate, and dietary fiber intake and risk of liver and biliary tract cancer in Western Europeans. Ann Oncol. 2013 Feb. 24(2). 543-553. https://www.ncbi.nlm.nih.gov/pubmed/23123507

[129] Moerman C, Bueno de Mesquita H., et al. Consumption of foods and micronutrients and the risk of cancer of the biliary tract. Prev Med. 1995 Nov. 24(6). 591-602.
https://www.ncbi.nlm.nih.gov/pubmed/8610083

[130] Glinsman W. Evaluation of health aspects of sugars contained in carbohydrate sweeteners. Report of Sugars Task Force. J Nutr 1986. P116. https://www.ncbi.nlm.nih.gov/pubmed/3543257

[131] Taubes G. Is sugar toxic? New York Times. Apr 13, 2011.
http://www.nytimes.com/2011/04/17/magazine/mag-17Sugar-t.html

[132] Yudkin J, Roddy J. Levels of dietary sucrose in patients with occlusive atherosclerotic disease. The Lancet 6(8). July 4, 1964. http://www.thelancet.com/journals/lancet/article/PIIS0140-6736(64)90003-0/abstract

[133] Yudkin J. Pure, White and Deadly. Orig. published 1972. Republished in 2012 Penguin Books.

[134] Dufty W. Sugar Blues. 1975 Warner Books.

[135] Appleton N. 141 reasons sugar ruins your health. NancyAppleton.com. https://nancyappleton.com/141-reasons-sugar-ruins-your-health/

[136] Appleton N. Lick The Sugar Habit. 1996. Avery.

[137] Taubes G. Is sugar toxic? New York Times. April 13, 2011. http://www.nytimes.com/2011/04/17/magazine/mag-17Sugar-t.html

[138] Taubes G. What if it's all been a big, fat lie? New York Times. July 7, 2002. http://www.nytimes.com/2002/07/07/magazine/what-if-it-s-all-been-a-big-fat-lie.html

[139] Taubes G. Why We Get Fat. Anchor Books. 2011.

[140] Pagliasotti M, Prach P, et al. Changes in insulin action, triglycerides and lipid composition during sucrose feeding in rats. Am J Physiol. 1996 Nov. 271(5 Pt 2) R1319-1326. https://www.ncbi.nlm.nih.gov/pubmed/8945970

[141] Jaggers J, Sui X, et al. Metabolic syndrome and risk of cancer mortality in men. Eur J Cancer 2009 Jul. 45(10). 1831-1838. https://www.ncbi.nlm.nih.gov/pmc/articles/PMC2700189/

[142] Foekens J, Prtengen H, et al. Insulin-like growth factor-1 receptors and insulin-like growth factor-1-like activity in human primary breast cancer. Cancer 1989 Jun 1. 63(11). 2139-2147. http://onlinelibrary.wiley.com/doi/10.1002/1097-0142(19890601)63:11%3C2139::AID-CNCR2820631112%3E3.0.CO%3B2-D/abstract

[143] Iwamura M, Sluss P, et al. Insulin-like growth factor-1: action and receptor characterization in human prostate cancer cell lines. Prostate.

1993. 22(3). 243-252.
http://onlinelibrary.wiley.com/doi/10.1002/pros.2990220307/abstract

[144] Kaiser U, Schardt C, et al. Expression of insulin-like growth factor receptors 1 and 2 in normal human lung and lung cancer. J Cancer Res Clin Oncol. 1993. 119(11). 665-668.
https://link.springer.com/article/10.1007/BF01215985

[145] Taubes G. Is sugar toxic? New York Times. Apr 13, 2011.
http://www.nytimes.com/2011/04/17/magazine/mag-17Sugar-t.html

[146] Warburg O, et al. Ueber den Stoffwechsel der Tumoren; Biochemische Zeitschrift. 152. pp.319-344. 1924. Reprinted in English in On Metabolism of Tumors. Constable. 1930.
https://www.ncbi.nlm.nih.gov/pmc/articles/PMC2140820/pdf/519.pdf

[147] Scheck A, Abdelwahab M, et al. The ketogenic diet for the treatment of glioma: insights from genetic profiling. Epilepsy Research. 100(3). Jul 2012. pp 327-337.
https://www.ncbi.nlm.nih.gov/pubmed/22019313

[148] Tisdale M, Brennan R, et al. A comparison of long-chain triglycerides and medium-chain triglycerides on weight loss and tumor size in a cachexia model. Br J Cancer. 1988 Nov. 58(5). 580-583.
https://www.ncbi.nlm.nih.gov/pmc/articles/PMC2246820/

[149] Freedland S, Mavropoulos J, et al. Carbohydrate restriction, prostate cancer growth, and the insulin-like growth factor axis. Prostate. 2008 Jan 1. 68(1). 11-19.
https://www.ncbi.nlm.nih.gov/pmc/articles/PMC3959866/

[150] Otto C, Kaemmerer U, et al. Growth of human gastric cancer cells in nude mice is delayed by a ketogenic diet supplemented with omega-3 fatty acids and medium-chain triglycerides. BMC Cancer. 2008 Apr 30. 8. 122. https://www.ncbi.nlm.nih.gov/pmc/articles/PMC2408928/

[151] Allen B, Bhatia S, et al. Ketogenic diets enhance oxidative stress and radio-chemotherapy responses in lung cancer xenografts. Clin Cancer Res. 2013 Jul 15. 19(4). 3905-3913.
https://www.ncbi.nlm.nih.gov/pmc/articles/PMC3954599/

[152] Schmidt M et al. Effects of a ketogenic diet on the quality of life in 16 patients with advanced cancer: a pilot trial. Nutr Metab. 2011 Jul 27. 8(1) 54. https://www.ncbi.nlm.nih.gov/pubmed/21794124

Chapter 9   Metabolic theory of cancer and common Misconceptions

[153] Israel B, Schaeffer W. Cytoplasmic suppression of malignancy. In Vitro Cell Dev Biol. 1987; 23:627-32.
https://link.springer.com/article/10.1007/BF02621071

[154] Israel B, Schaeffer W. Cytoplasmic mediation of malignancy. In Vitro Cell Dev Biol. 1988; 24:487-90.
https://www.ncbi.nlm.nih.gov/pubmed/3372452

[155] Shay J, Werbin H. Cytoplasmic suppression of tumorigenicity in reconstructed mouse cells. Cancer Res. 1988; 48: 830-33.
http://cancerres.aacrjournals.org/content/canres/48/4/830.full.pdf

[156] Shay, J, Liu Y, Werbin H. Cytoplasmic suppression of tumor progression in reconstituted cells. Somat Cell Mol Genet. 1988; 14:345-50.
[157] Christofferson T. Tripping Over The Truth. Create Space Independent Publishing Platform. 2014.
[158] Salk J, Fox E, et al. Mutational heterogenicity in human cancers: origin and consequences. Annu Rev Pathol. 2010; 5:51-75.
https://www.ncbi.nlm.nih.gov/pubmed/19743960

[159] Wu J, Fackler M, et al. Heterogeneity of breast cancer metastases: comparison of therapeutic target expression and promoter methylation between primary tumors and their multifocal metastases. Clin Cancer Res. 2008; 14:1938-46.
https://www.ncbi.nlm.nih.gov/pubmed/18381931

[160] Campbell P, Yachida S. et al. The patterns and dynamics of genomic instability in metastatic pancreatic cancer. Nature: 2010; 467: 1109-13. https://www.ncbi.nlm.nih.gov/pubmed/20981101

[161] Ohgaki H, Kleiheus P. Genetic alterations and signaling pathways in the evolution of gliomas. Cancer Sci. 2009; 100:2235-41.
https://www.ncbi.nlm.nih.gov/pubmed/19737147

[162] Warburg O. On respiratory impairment in cancer cells. Science. 1956, 124(3215): 269-70.

[163] Christofferson T. Tripping Over The Truth. Op cit.

[164] Seyfried T. Cancer as a Metabolic Disease. Wiley. 2012.

[165] Christofferson T. op cit.

[166] US National Library of Medicine. The Rosalind Franklin papers. Profiles in Science. National Institutes of Health, Bethesda, MD. www.profiles.nlm.nih.gov.

Chapter 10   The problem with chemotherapy

[167] Weintraub P. Integrative oncology: a healthier way to fight cancer. Experience Life. 2013 May. https://experiencelife.com/article/integrative-oncology-a-healthier-way-to-fight-cancer/

[168] Mukherjee S. The Emperor of All Maladies: A Biography of Cancer. Scribner. 2011 Aug.

Chapter 11   How did most doctors get trapped into disease management rather than health counseling?

[169] Christofferson T. op cit.

[170] Christofferson T. op cit.

[171] Levinson D. Consultations in Medicare: Coding & Reimbursement. Dept of Health and Human Services, Office of Inspector General. Mar 2006. https://oig.hhs.gov/oei/reports/oei-09-02-00030.pdf

[172] Moss E, Hollingworth J, et al. The role of CA-125 in clinical practice. J Clin Pathol. Mar 2005. 58(3). 308-312. https://www.ncbi.nlm.nih.gov/pubmed/15735166

[173] Quoted in www.naturopathicstandards.org.

[174] Bollinger T The Truth About Cancer. Hay House. 2016.

[175] Fitzgerald, Benedict, "A Report to the Senate Interstate Commerce Committee on The Need for Investigation of Cancer Research Organizations," Congressional Record 1953: A5350. https://archive.org/stream/FitzgeraldReportCarnegieRockerfellerTheA MAAndTheBirthOfModernMedicineYouTube/fitzgerald report Report to the Senate Interstate Commerce Committee on the Need for Investigation of Cancer Research Organizations_djvu.txt

[176] Ibid.

[177] Getzendanner S., Permanent Injunction Order Against AMA. JAMA 1988. 259(1):81. https://jamanetwork.com/journals/jama/article-abstract/370078

[178] Federal Trade Commission. The Anti-Trust Laws. https://www.ftc.gov/tips-advice/competition-guidance/guide-antitrust-laws/antitrust-laws

[179] George Washington University. Power in numbers: Lobbyists have Congress covered. Face The Facts USA. Jan 2013. http://www.facethefactsusa.org/facts/power-numbers-lobbyists-have-congress-covered

[180] Cornell Law School. 21 US Code Chapter 9. Federal Food, Drug and Cosmetic Act. 1938. https://www.law.cornell.edu/uscode/text/21/chapter-9

Chapter 12   Four major dietary mistakes made by most cancer patients

[181] USDA Cooperative Extension. On average, how many pounds of corn make one pound of beef? Oct 7, 2008. http://articles.extension.org/pages/35850/on-average-how-many-pounds-of-corn-make-one-pound-of-beef-assuming-an-all-grain-diet-from-background

[182] Boehrer K. This is how much water it takes to make your favorite foods.www.huffingtonpost.com. Apr 13,2015.

[183] Cordain L. The Paleo Diet. John Wiley & Sons. Dec.7, 2010.

[184] Winters SF, Loebel F, et al. Role of ketogenic metabolic therapy in malignant glioma: a systematic review. Crit Rev Oncol Hematol. 2017 Apr. 112:41-58. https://www.ncbi.nlm.nih.gov/pubmed/28325264

[185] Klement RJ. Beneficial effects of ketogenic diets for cancer patients: a realist review with focus on evidence and confirmation. Med Oncol. 2017 Aug. 34(8): 132. https://www.ncbi.nlm.nih.gov/pubmed/28653283

[186] United States Department of Agriculture (USDA).

[187] Wise D DeBerardinis R, et al. Myc regulates a transcriptional program that stimulates mitochondrial glutaminolysis and leads to glutamine addiction. Proc Nat Acad Sci 2008 Dec. 105(48):18782-7. doi: 10.1073/pnas.0810199105 https://www.ncbi.nlm.nih.gov/pubmed/19033189

[188] LawrenceT, Gilroy D. Chronic inflammation: a failure of resolution? Int J Exp Pathol. 2007; 88:85-94. https://www.ncbi.nlm.nih.gov/pubmed/17408451

[189] Seyfried T. op cit. p.309.

[190] Seyfried T. op cit. p. 380.

Chapter 14   Exercise and oxygen

[191] American College of Sports Medicine. http://www.acsm.org/about-acsm/media-room/acsm-in-the-news/2011/08/01/acsm-aha-support-federal-physical-activity-guidelines.

[192] Berryman J. Exercise is medicine: a historical perspective. Curr Sports Med Rep. 2010 Jul-Aug. 9(4) 195-201. https://www.ncbi.nlm.nih.gov/pubmed/20622536

[193] Oaklander M. The new science of exercise. Time: The Science of Exercise. http://time.com/4475628/the-new-science-of-exercise/

[194] Ibid.

[195] Brand R. Biographical sketch: Otto Heinrich Warburg, PhD, MD. Clinical Orthopaedics and Related Research. 2010 Nov. 468(11): 2831-32. www.ncbi.nlm.nih.gov/pmc/articles/PMC2947689.

[196] DeClerck K, Elble RC. The role of hypoxia and acidosis in promoting metastasis and resistance to chemotherapy. Front Biosci (Landmark Ed) 2010;15:213–225.
https://www.ncbi.nlm.nih.gov/pubmed/20036816

[197] Sweet F, Kao M, et al. Ozone selectively inhibits growth of human cancer cells. Science. 1980. 209: 931-933.
https://www.ncbi.nlm.nih.gov/pubmed/7403859

[198] Efrati S, Golan H, et al. Hyperbaric oxygen therapy can diminish fibromyalgia syndrome. Plos One. 2015; 10(5): e0127012.
http://journals.plos.org/plosone/article?id=10.1371/journal.pone.0127012

Chapter 15   Vitamin C

[199] Chen Q, Espey M, Krishna M, et al. Pharmacologic ascorbic acid concentrations selectively kill cancer cells: action as a pro-drug to deliver hydrogen peroxide to tissues. Proc Natl Acad Sci. 2005 Sep; 102(38): 13604-09.
https://www.ncbi.nlm.nih.gov/pubmed/16157892

[200] Bonuccelli G, de Francesco E, et al. NADH autofluorescence, a new metabolic biomarker for cancer stem cells: identification of Vitamin C and CAPE as natural products targeting "stemness." Oncotarget. 2017. 8(13). 20667-20678.
http://www.impactjournals.com/oncotarget/index.php?journal=oncotarget&page=article&op=view&path%5B%5D=15400&path%5B%5D=49203

[201] Cimmino L, Dolgalev I, et al. Restoration of TET2 function blocks aberrant self-renewal and leukemia progression. Cell. 170(6). 1079-95. http://www.cell.com/cell/fulltext/S0092-8674(17)30868-1

[202] Science Daily. Vitamin C may encourage blood cancer stem cells to die. Aug 2017.
https://www.sciencedaily.com/releases/2017/08/170817141722.htm

[203] Science Daily. Vitamin C effective in targeting cancer stem cells. Mar 2017.
https://www.sciencedaily.com/releases/2017/03/170308083940.htm

Chapter 16   Sodium bicarbonate

[204] Estrella V. Acidity generated by the tumor microenvironment drives local invasion. Cancer Res. Mar 2013.
https://www.ncbi.nlm.nih.gov/pubmed/23288510

[205] Silva A et al. The potential role of synthetic buffers in reducing intratumoral extracellular pH and acid-mediated invasion. Cancer Res. Mar 2009. https://www.ncbi.nlm.nih.gov/pubmed/19276380.

[206] Robey I. Bicarbonate increases tumor pH and inhibits spontaneous metastases. Cancer Res. Mar 2009.
https://www.ncbi.nlm.nih.gov/pubmed/19276390

[207] Fischer, K, Hoffmann P, et al. Inhibitory effect of tumor cell–derived lactic acid on human T cells. Blood 109.9 (2007): 3812-3819
https://www.ncbi.nlm.nih.gov/pubmed/17255361

[208] Beckert, S, Farrahi, F, et al. Lactate stimulates endothelial cell migration. Wound repair and regeneration 14.3 (2006): 321-324.
https://www.ncbi.nlm.nih.gov/pubmed/16808811

[209] Estrella V. Op cit.
https://www.ncbi.nlm.nih.gov/pubmed/23288510

[210] Simoncini, Tullio. Cancer is a Fungus: A Revolution in Tumor Therapy. 2nd ed., Edizione Lamte. 2007.

[211] Potassium bicarbonate (073508) and Sodium bicarbonate (073505) Fact Sheet *United States Environmental Protection Agency*. Updated 17 February 2011. Retrieved 25 November 2011.

Chapter 17   Vitamin A

[212] Ries J Blasiu A. Vitamin A therapy of carcinomata. Munch Med. 1952. https://www.ncbi.nlm.nih.gov/pubmed/12993091

[213] Li C, Imai M, et al. Effects of pre- and post-administration of vitamin A on the growth of refractory cancers in xenograft mice. Biol Pharm. Apr 2017. https://www.ncbi.nlm.nih.gov/pubmed/28100867

[214] Jones C, Sly L, et al. Retinol and beta-carotene concentrations in skin, papillomas and carcinomas, liver and serum of mice fed retinoic acid or beta-carotene to suppress skin tumor formation. Nutr Cancer. 1994. https://www.ncbi.nlm.nih.gov/pubmed/7910392

[215] Ponnamperuma R, Shimizu Y, et al. Beta-carotene fails to act as a tumor promoter, induces RAR expression, and prevents carcinoma formation in a two-stage model of skin carcinogenesis in male Sencar mice. Nutr Cancer. 2000.
https://www.ncbi.nlm.nih.gov/pubmed/10965524.

[216] Bhatia A, Lee J, et al. Double-blind, randomized phase 3 trial of low-dose 13-cis retinoic acid in the prevention of second primaries in head and neck cancer. Cancer. Aug 2017.
https://www.ncbi.nlm.nih.gov/pubmed/28786105

[217] Toma S, Bonelli L, et al. 13-ciis retinoic acid in head and neck cancer chemoprevention: results of a randomized trial from the Italian Head and Neck Chemoprevention Study Group. Oncol Rep. Jun 2004. https://www.ncbi.nlm.nih.gov/pubmed/15138569.

[218] Sobotka R, Capoun O, et al. Prognostic importance of vitamins A, E and retinol-binding protein 4 in renal cell carcinoma patients. Anticancer Res. Jul 2017.
https://www.ncbi.nlm.nih.gov/pubmed/28668878.

[219] Li C, Imai M et al. Inhibitory effects of retinol are greater than retinoic acid on the growth and adhesion of human refractory cancer cells. Biol Pharm. Jan 2016.
https://www.ncbi.nlm.nih.gov/pubmed/26822412

[220] Tang J, Wang R, et al. Vitamin A and risk of bladder cancer: a meta-analysis of epidemiological studies. World J Surg Oncol. Apr 2014. https://www.ncbi.nlm.nih.gov/pmc/articles/PMC4030017/

[221] Suri S, Kumar D, et al. Dietary deficiency of vitamin A among rural children: a community-based survey using a food-frequency

questionnaire. Natl Med J India. Mar 2017.
https://www.ncbi.nlm.nih.gov/pubmed/28816210

[222] Harris E, Loewenstein J, Azar D. Vitamin A deficiency and its effects on the eye. Int. Ophthalmol Clin 1998; 38:155-61.
[223] Spits Y, DeLaey J, Leroy B. Rapid recovery of night blindness due to obesity surgery after vitamin A repletion therapy. Br J Ophthalmol. Apr 2004. https://www.ncbi.nlm.nih.gov/pmc/articles/PMC1772100/

[224] Uray I, Dmitrovsky E. Retinoids and rexinoids in cancer prevention: from laboratory to clinic. Semin Oncol. Feb 2016. 43(1): 49-64. https://www.ncbi.nlm.nih.gov/pmc/articles/PMC4789177/

[225] Okayasu I, Hana K, et al. Vitamin A inhibits development of dextran-sulfate sodium-induced colitis and colon cancer in a mouse model. Biomed Res Int. May 2016.
https://www.ncbi.nlm.nih.gov/pmc/articles/PMC4889797/

[226] Idres N et al. Granulocytic differentiation of human NB4 Promyelocytic leukemia cells induced by all-trans retinoic acid metabolites. Cancer Res. Jan 2001; 61(2): 700-705.
https://www.ncbi.nlm.nih.gov/pubmed/11212271

[227] Nagy L, Thomazy V, et al. Activation of retinoid X receptors induces apoptosis in HL-60 cell lines. Mol Cell Biol. Jul 1995. 15(7): 3540-51. https://www.ncbi.nlm.nih.gov/pubmed/7791761

[228] Audette M, Page M. Growth modification of normal and tumor cell lines with retinol. Cancer Detect Prev. 1983; 6(6): 497-505.
https://www.ncbi.nlm.nih.gov/pubmed/6661740

[229] Botilsrud M, Holmberg I et al. Effect of retinoids and 1,25(OH)2 vitamin D3 bound to their plasma transport proteins on growth and differentiation of HL-60 cells. Scand J Clin Lab Invest. May 1990; 50(3):309-17. https://www.ncbi.nlm.nih.gov/pubmed/2353161

[230] Halter S, Fraker L, et al. Selective isolation of human breast carcinoma cells resistant to the growth-inhibitory effects of retinol. Nutr Cancer 1990; 14(1):43-56.
https://www.ncbi.nlm.nih.gov/pubmed/2367235

[231] Meyskens F, Fuller B. Characterization of the effects of different retinoids on the growth and differentiation of human melanoma cell

line and selected subclones. Cancer Res. Jul 1980. 40(7):2194-6.
https://www.ncbi.nlm.nih.gov/pubmed/6770995

[232] Culine S, Kramear A, et al. Phase II study of all-trans-retinoic acid administered intermittently for hormone-refractory prostate cancer. J Urol. Jan 1999. 161(1): 173-75.
https://www.ncbi.nlm.nih.gov/pubmed/9025776

[233] Fazely F, Ledinko N, et al. Inhibition by retinoids of in vitro invasive ability of human lung carcinoma cells. Anticancer Res Nov Dec 1988: 8(6): 1387-91.
https://www.ncbi.nlm.nih.gov/pubmed/2905883

[234] Culine S, Kramear A. ibid.
https://www.ncbi.nlm.nih.gov/pubmed/9025776

[235] Conley B, Egorin M et al. Phase I clinical trial of all-trans retinoic acid with correlation of its pharmacokinetics and pharmacodynamics. Cancer Chemother Pharmacol. 1997. 39(4) 291-99.
https://www.ncbi.nlm.nih.gov/pubmed/9025769

Chapter 18   Vitamin D

[236] Giovannucci E. The epidemiology of vitamin D and cancer incidence and mortality: a review. Cancer Causes Control. 2005 Mar; 16(2): 83-95. https://www.ncbi.nlm.nih.gov/pubmed/15868450

[237] Wei M, Garland C, et al. Vitamin D and prevention of colorectal adenoma: a meta-analysis. Cancer Epidemiol Biomarkers Prev. 2008 Nov; 17(11): 2958-69.
https://www.ncbi.nlm.nih.gov/pubmed/18990737

[238] Garland C, Gorham E, et al. Vitamin D for cancer prevention: global perspective. Ann Epidem 2009 Jul;19(7):468-83.
https://www.ncbi.nlm.nih.gov/pubmed/19523595

[239] Giovannucci E. Vitamin D and cancer incidence in the Harvard cohorts. Ann Epidem. 2009 Feb 19(2): 84-8.
https://www.ncbi.nlm.nih.gov/pubmed/18291673

[240] De Smedt J, Van Kelst S, et al. Vitamin D supplementation in cutaneous malignant melanoma outcome (ViDMe): a randomized controlled trial. BMC Cancer. Aug 2017. 17(1): 562.
https://www.ncbi.nlm.nih.gov/pubmed/28835228

[241] Vahedpoor Z, Jamilian M, et al. Effects of long-term vitamin D supplementation on regression and metabolic status of cervical intraepithelial neoplasia: a randomized, double-blind, placebo-controlled trial. Horm Cancer. Feb 2017. 8(1): 58-67.
https://www.ncbi.nlm.nih.gov/pubmed/28050798

[242] Jarrard D, Konety B, et al. Phase IIa, randomized placebo-controlled trial of single high dose cholecalciferol (vitamin D3) and daily genistein (G-2535) versus double placebo in men with early stage prostate cancer undergoing prostatectomy. Am J Clin Exp Urol. Sept 2016. 20;4(2): 17-27.
https://www.ncbi.nlm.nih.gov/pubmed/27766277.

[243] Bostick RM. Effects of supplemental vitamin D and calcium on normal colon tissue and circulating biomarkers of risk for colorectal neoplasms. J Steroid Biochem Mol Biol. Apr 2015, 148:86-95.
https://www.ncbi.nlm.nih.gov/pubmed/25597952

[244] Fedirko V, Bostick R, et al. Effects of supplemental vitamin D and calcium on oxidative DNA damage marker in normal colorectal mucosa: a randomized clinical trial. Cancer Epidemiol Biomarkers Prev. Jan 2010. 19(1): 280-91.
https://www.ncbi.nlm.nih.gov/pubmed/20056649

[245] Schumann, S, Ewigman B. Double-dose vitamin D lowers cancer risk in women over 55. J Fam Pract. Nov 2007. 56(11): 907-910.
https://www.ncbi.nlm.nih.gov/pmc/articles/PMC4294452/

[246] Lappe J, Travers-Gustafson D. Vitamin D and calcium supplementation reduces cancer risk: results of a randomized trial. Am J Clin Nutr. Jun 2007. 85(6):1586-91.
https://www.ncbi.nlm.nih.gov/pubmed/17556697

[247] Brunner R, Wactawski-Wende J, et al. The effect of calcium plus vitamin D on risk for invasive cancer: results of the Women's Health Initiative (WHI) calcium plus vitamin D randomized clinical trial. Nutr Cancer. 2011. 63(6): 827-41.
https://www.ncbi.nlm.nih.gov/pubmed/21774589

[248] Li M, Li L, et al. 1,25-dihydroxyvitamin D3 suppresses gastric cancer cell growth through VDR- and mutant p53-mediated induction of p21. Life Sci. Jun 2017. 179: 88-97.

[249] Pourgholami M, Akhter J. In vitro and in vivo inhibition of liver cancer cells by 1,25-dihydroxyvitamin D3. Cancer Lett. Apr 2000. 151(1):97-102. https://www.ncbi.nlm.nih.gov/pubmed/10766428

[250] Saez S, Falette N, et al. 1,25(OH)2D3 modulation of mammary tumor cell growth in vitro and in vivo. William L. McGuire Memorial Symposium. Breast Cancer Res Treat. 1993. 27(1-2):69-81. https://www.ncbi.nlm.nih.gov/pubmed/8260731

[251] Shen M, Yen A. Nicotinamide cooperates with retinoic acid and 1,25 dihydroxyvitamin D(3) to regulate cell differentiation and cell cycle arrest of human myeloblastic leukemia cells. Oncology 2009; 76(2): 91-100. https://www.ncbi.nlm.nih.gov/pubmed/19127080

[252] Kizildag S, Ates H, et al. Treatment of K562 cells with 1,25 dihydroxyvitamin D(3) induces distinct alterations in the expression of apoptosis-related genes BCL-2, BAX, BCL(XL) and p21. Ann Hematol. 2009 May 28. https://www.ncbi.nlm.nih.gov/pubmed/19475409

[253] Wu W, Zhang X, et al. 1alpha, 25 dihydroxyvitamin D(3) anti-proliferative actions involving vitamin D receptor-mediated activation of MAPK pathways and AP-1/p21 (waf1) upregulation in human osteosarcoma. Cancer Lett. 2007 Aug 28. 254(1): 75-86. https://www.ncbi.nlm.nih.gov/pubmed/17412493

[254] Fujioka T, Suzuki Y, et al. Prevention of renal cell carcinoma by active vitamin D(3). World J Surg. 2000 Oct; 24(10): 1205-10. https://www.ncbi.nlm.nih.gov/pubmed/11071463

[255] Bao B, Yao J, et al. 1alpha, 25-dihydroxyvitamin D3 suppresses interleukin-8-mediated prostate cancer cell angiogenesis. Carcinogenesis. 2006 Sep; 27(9): 1883-93. https://www.ncbi.nlm.nih.gov/pubmed/16624828

[256] Chung I, Han G, et al. Role of Vitamin D receptor in the antiproliferative effects of calcitriol in tumor-derived endothelial cells and tumor angiogenesis in vivo. Cancer Res. 2009 Feb 1; 69(3). 967-75. https://www.ncbi.nlm.nih.gov/pubmed/19141646

[257] Yudoh K, Matsuno H, et al. 1alpha, 25-dihydroxyvitamin D3 inhibits in vitro invasiveness through the extracellular matrix and in vivo pulmonary metastasis of mouse melanoma. J Lab Clin Med. 1999 Feb 133(2): 120-8.
https://www.ncbi.nlm.nih.gov/pubmed/9989763

[258] Defacue H, Commes T. Synergistic differentiation of U937 cells by all-trans retinoic acid and 1 alpha, 25-dihydroxyvitamin D3 is associated with the expression of retinoid X receptor alpha. Biochem Biophys Res Commun. Aug 1994. 203(1):272-80.
https://www.ncbi.nlm.nih.gov/pubmed/8074666

[259] Blutt S, Allegretto E. 1,25-dihydroxyvitamin D3 and 9-cis-retinoic acid act synergistically to inhibit the growth of LNCaP prostate cells and cause accumulation of cells in G1. Endocrinology. Apr 1997. 138(4):1491-7. https://www.ncbi.nlm.nih.gov/pubmed/9075707

[260] Verstuyf A, Mathieu C. Differentiation induction of human leukemia cells (HL60) by a combination of 1,25-dihydroxyitamin D3 and retinoic acid (all trans or 9-cis). J Steroid Biochem Mol Biol. Jun 1995. 53(1-6):431-41.
https://www.ncbi.nlm.nih.gov/pubmed/7626492

[261] Fossella FV. Docetaxel for previously treated non-small-cell lung cancer. Oncology. Jun 2002. 16 (6 Suppl 6): 45-51.
https://www.ncbi.nlm.nih.gov/pubmed/12108897

Chapter 19 Randomized, placebo-controlled trials of nutrients against cancer

[262] Shepherd F, Dancey J, et al. Prospective randomized trial of docetaxel versus best supportive care in patients with non-small-cell lung cancer previously treated with platinum-based chemotherapy. J Clin Oncol, 18(10) 2095-2103. May 2000. Pub Med 10811675.
https://www.ncbi.nlm.nih.gov/labs/pubmed/10811675-prospective-randomized-trial-of-docetaxel-versus-best-supportive-care-in-patients-with-non-small-cell-lung-cancer-previously-treated-with-platinum-based-chemotherapy/

[263] Naturopathic Cancer Society. Which cancer are you researching? www.NatOnco.org.

[264] Taylor P, Li B, et al. Prevention of esophageal cancer: the nutrition intervention trials in Linxian, China. Linxian Nutrition Intervention Trials Study Group. Cancer Res. Apr 1994. 1;54(7 Suppl): 2029s-2031s. https://www.ncbi.nlm.nih.gov/pubmed/8137333

[265] Greenwald P, Anderson D, et al. Clinical trials of vitamin and mineral supplements for cancer prevention. American Journal of Clinical Nutrition. Jan 2007. 85(1); 3145-3175. http://ajcn.nutrition.org/content/85/1/314S.full#ref-21

[266] Zhang S, Moore S et al. Folate, vitamin B6, multivitamin supplements and colorectal cancer risk in women. Am J Epidemiol 2006; 163:108-15. https://www.ncbi.nlm.nih.gov/pmc/articles/PMC1363749/

[267] Vahedpoor Z, Jamilian M, et al. Effects of long-term vitamin D supplementation on regression and metabolic status of cervical intraepithelial neoplasia: a randomized, double-blind, placebo-controlled trial. Horm Cancer. Feb 2017. 8(1): 58-67. https://www.ncbi.nlm.nih.gov/pubmed/28050798

[268] Bostick RM. Effects of supplemental vitamin D and calcium on normal colon tissue and circulating biomarkers of risk for colorectal neoplasms. J Steroid Biochem Mol Biol. Apr 2015, 148:86-95. https://www.ncbi.nlm.nih.gov/pubmed/25597952

[269] Fedirko V, Bostick R, et al. Effects of supplemental vitamin D and calcium on oxidative DNA damage marker in normal colorectal mucosa: a randomized clinical trial. Cancer Epidemiol Biomarkers Prev. Jan 2010. 19(1): 280-91. https://www.ncbi.nlm.nih.gov/pubmed/20056649

[270] De Smedt J, Van Kelst S, et al. Vitamin D supplementation in cutaneous malignant melanoma outcome (ViDMe): a randomized controlled trial. BMC Cancer. Aug 2017. 17(1): 562. https://www.ncbi.nlm.nih.gov/pubmed/28835228

[271] Jarrard D, Konety B, et al. Phase IIa, randomized placebo-controlled trial of single high dose cholecalciferol (vitamin D3) and daily genistein (G-2535) versus double placebo in men with early stage prostate cancer undergoing prostatectomy. Am J Clin Exp Urol. Sept 2016. 20;4(2): 17-27. https://www.ncbi.nlm.nih.gov/pubmed/27766277.

[272] Schumann, S, Ewigman B. Double-dose vitamin D lowers cancer risk in women over 55. J Fam Pract. Nov 2007. 56(11): 907-910.
https://www.ncbi.nlm.nih.gov/pmc/articles/PMC4294452/

[273] Lappe J, Travers-Gustafson D. Vitamin D and calcium supplementation reduces cancer risk: results of a randomized trial. Am J Clin Nutr. Jun 2007. 85(6):1586-91.
https://www.ncbi.nlm.nih.gov/pubmed/17556697

[274] Brunner R, Wactawski-Wende J, et al. The effect of calcium plus vitamin D on risk for invasive cancer: results of the Women's Health Initiative (WHI) calcium plus vitamin D randomized clinical trial. Nutr Cancer. 2011. 63(6): 827-41.
https://www.ncbi.nlm.nih.gov/pubmed/21774589

[275] Li M, Li L, et al. 1,25-dihydroxyvitamin D3 suppresses gastric cancer cell growth through VDR- and mutant p53-mediated induction of p21. Life Sci. Jun 2017. 179: 88-97.
https://www.ncbi.nlm.nih.gov/pubmed/?term=1%2C25-dihydroxyvitamin+D3+suppresses+gastric+cancer+cell+growth+through+VDR-+and+mutant+p53-mediated+induction+of+p21.++Life+Sci

[276] Pourgholami M, Akhter J. In vitro and in vivo inhibition of liver cancer cells by 1,25-dihydroxyvitamin D3. Cancer Lett. Apr 2000. 151(1):97-102. https://www.ncbi.nlm.nih.gov/pubmed/10766428

[277] Saez S, Falette N, et al. 1,25(OH)2D3 modulation of mammary tumor cell growth in vitro and in vivo. William L. McGuire Memorial Symposium. Breast Cancer Res Treat. 1993. 27(1-2):69-81.
https://www.ncbi.nlm.nih.gov/pubmed/8260731

[278] Defacue H, Commes T. Synergistic differentiation of U937 cells by all-trans retinoic acid and 1 alpha, 25-dihydroxyvitamin D3 is associated with the expression of retinoid X receptor alpha. Biochem Biophys Res Commun. Aug 1994. 203(1):272-80.
https://www.ncbi.nlm.nih.gov/pubmed/8074666

[279] Blutt S, Allegretto E. 1,25-dihydroxyvitamin D3 and 9-cis-retinoic acid act synergistically to inhibit the growth of LNCaP prostate cells and cause accumulation of cells in G1. Endocrinology. Apr 1997. 138(4):1491-7. https://www.ncbi.nlm.nih.gov/pubmed/9075707

[280] Verstuyf A, Mathieu C. Differentiation induction of human leukemia cells (HL60) by a combination of 1,25-dihydroxyitamin D3 and retinoic acid (all trans or 9-cis). J Steroid Biochem Mol Biol. Jun 1995. 53(1-6):431-41.
https://www.ncbi.nlm.nih.gov/pubmed/7626492

Chapter 20   Randomized, placebo-controlled trials of herbs against cancer

[281] Citronberg J, Bostick R, et al. Effects of ginger supplementation on cell-cycle biomarkers in the normal-appearing colonic mucosa of patients at increased risk for colorectal cancer: results from a pilot, randomized, and controlled trial. Cancer Prev Res (Phila). Apr 2013 6(4). 271-81. https://www.ncbi.nlm.nih.gov/pubmed/23303903

[282] Susak Y, Zemskov S, et al. Comparison of chemotherapy and X-ray therapy with Ukrain monotherapy for colorectal cancer. Drugs Exp Clin Res. 1996; 22:115-22.
https://www.ncbi.nlm.nih.gov/pubmed/8899313

[283] Zemskov S, Procopchuk O, et al. Ukrain (NSC 631570) in the treatment of pancreas cancer. Drugs Exp Clin Res. 2000; 26(5-6): 179-90. https://www.ncbi.nlm.nih.gov/pubmed/11345025

[284] Uglyanitsa K, Nefyodov L, et al. Comparative evaluation of the efficiency of various Ukrain doses in the combined treatment of breast cancer. Report 1. Clinical aspects of Ukrain application. Drugs Exp Clin Res. 2000; 26(5-6). 223-30.
https://www.ncbi.nlm.nih.gov/pubmed/11345029

[285] Ernst E, Schmidt K. Ukrain – a new cancer cure? A systematic review of randomized clinical trials. BMC Cancer. 2005; 5:69.
https://www.ncbi.nlm.nih.gov/pmc/articles/PMC1180428/#B120

[286] Van Die M, Bone K, et al. Phytotherapeutic interventions in the management of biochemically recurrent prostate cancer: a systematic review of randomised trials. BJU Int. Apr 2016; 117 Suppl 4:17-34.
https://www.ncbi.nlm.nih.gov/pubmed/26898239

[287] Thomas R, Williams M, et al. A double-blind, placebo-controlled randomized trial evaluating the effect of a polyphenol-rich whole food supplement on PSA progression in men with prostate cancer – the UK

NCRN Pomi-T study. Prostate Cancer Prostatic Disease. Jun 2014; 17(2): 180-6. https://www.ncbi.nlm.nih.gov/pubmed/24614693

[288] Wang S, Wang Q, et al. Astragalus-containing Traditional Chinese Medicine, with and without prescription based on syndrome differentiation, combined with chemotherapy for advanced non-small-cell lung cancer: a systemic review and meta-analysis. Curr. Oncol. Jun 2016; 23(3).e: 188-95. https://www.ncbi.nlm.nih.gov/pubmed/27330356

Chapter 21   Hyperthermia

[289] NIH National Cancer Institute. Hyperthermia in cancer treatment. Aug 2011. https://www.cancer.gov/about-cancer/treatment/types/surgery/hyperthermia-fact-sheet

[290] Van der Zee J. Heating the patient: a promising approach? Ann Oncol. Aug 2002. 13(8). 1173-84. https://www.ncbi.nlm.nih.gov/pubmed/12181239

[291] Hildebrandt B, Wust P, et al. The cellular and molecular basis of hyperthermia. Crit Rev Oncol Hematol. Jul 2002. 43(1): 33-56. https://www.ncbi.nlm.nih.gov/pubmed/12098606

[292] Falk M, Issels R, et al. Hyperthermia in oncology. Int J Hyperthermia. Jan-Feb 2001. (17)1:1-18. https://www.ncbi.nlm.nih.gov/pubmed/11212876

[293] Op. cit. NIH National Cancer Institute. Hyperthermia in cancer treatment. https://www.cancer.gov/about-cancer/treatment/types/surgery/hyperthermia-fact-sheet

[294] Ernst E, Pecho E, et al. Regular sauna bathing and the incidence of common colds. Ann Med. 22.4. (1990): 225-27. https://www.ncbi.nlm.nih.gov/pubmed/2248758

Chapter 22   Opposition to natural medicine

[295] Hanson M. A hundred and fifty years of misuse of mercury and dental amalgam – still a lesson to learn. http://art-bin.com/art/hanson_en.html.

Made in the USA
Las Vegas, NV
27 January 2023

66333120R00163